MW01028607

Becky Chambers has introduce
combination of homeopathy ar
better for healing than each of .
the book; the combination may work for you. Even scientific
materialists should be interested because Chambers presents a
new nanotechnology-based theory in support of homeopathy
along with older theories.

—AMIT GOSWAMI, PhD,
quantum physicist and author
of *The Quantum Doctor* and *Quantum Economics*

Being a one-trick pony, I am always impressed when an
accomplished homeopath takes on the task of mastering
a second field of healing. Like Whitmont (homeopathy
and Jungian thought), Helms (homeopathy and TCM),
and Nerman (homeopathy and cranial osteopathy),
Becky Chambers has written a text which expands our
understanding of two fields. Kudos.

—ROGER MORRISON, MD,
author of *Desktop Guide to Keynotes
and Confirmatory Symptoms*

This book presents ideas that are novel and new—it is a must
read for the large number of people who have turned toward
holistic medicine. The concept of mixing energy stimulation
or modulation into a therapeutic regimen is very relevant in
clinical practice. I highly recommend this book.

—STEPHEN HOLT, MD, DSc, ND,
Distinguished Professor of Medicine Emeritus

Becky Chambers, in her person—as she has lived her life—and in writing her new book, *Homeopathy Plus Whole Body Vibration: Combining Two Energy Medicines Ignites Healing,* has begun the work of bringing together two fields not usually connected. This is a book that I, as a Jungian analyst, will recommend to many in my depth psychology practice where we continuously probe the interface of body and soul, soma and psyche. This book helps all of us understand how the "releasing" of symptomatic issues takes place through many layers manifest in body and psyche. Her work also helps us understand how to bring about healing.

—THOMAS J. KAPACINSKAS, JD, NCPsyA, past president, Chicago Society of Jungian Analysts

I've been a big believer in energy medicine and healing modalities for over twenty years and have incorporated many of them in my own healthcare regimen. In today's world, we are bombarded on a regular basis with advertisements for pharmaceuticals to take care of a whole host of symptoms—and, of course, that's after you listen to or read a long list of possible side effects (including death). More than ever, many of us are interested in living healthy, vibrant lives—especially as we age. It's past time that we investigate healthcare solutions used by physicians all over the world that are powerful, gentle, and have no side effects. In *Homeopathy Plus Whole Body Vibration,* Becky Chambers introduces us to two therapies that are powerful on their own. Combined, they offer a synergistic healing force that can rock your world—your body, your mind, and your spirit. Read some of the real-life healing journeys that Chambers shares. If what you've been doing isn't working and/or if you're ready to optimize your health and have your energy soar, this could be for you.

—ANN QUASMAN, chief fulfillment officer and creator of *Conscious Conversations Café* on WomanTalk Live Radio, www.WomanTalkLive.com

Homeopathy Plus Whole Body Vibration describes in detail how two very effective, energy-based treatments can be combined to aid in the detoxification and realignment of our energy body. Many of our current health problems are due to toxic chemical and emotional overload. Homeopathy is one of the most effective methods for detoxification. Combined with WBV, a powerful physical technique to help detoxification, they produce a very effective synergistic program for regaining your health.

—SUSAN E. KOLB, MD, FACS, ABIHM,
plastic surgeon, author of *The Naked Truth about Breast Implants,* and host of the *Temple of Health* radio show

In highly readable fashion, Becky Chambers introduces and explains the transformational impact of the combined use of homeopathy and whole body vibration and the research that supports both. Recognized in Europe (and in the US as recently as the late nineteenth century) as a gentle and effective treatment for a variety of ailments, homeopathy fell victim to the political alliance of the AMA and pharmaceutical companies [in the US]. As a daughter of a physician, I was raised with a great distrust of alternative medicine. Yet the combination of homeopathy and WBV has begun to alleviate chronic symptoms that numerous physicians have been unable to fix.

—TRACY WALLACH, PhD,
expert in group, organizational, and socio-political systems

Homeopathy Plus Whole Body Vibration

Combining Two
Energy Medicines
Ignites Healing

Becky Chambers

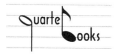
Quarter Books

Cover design by Darryl Khalil
Interior design by Steve Amarillo
Author photo by Miranda Loud

Book production by
Quartet Books
Charlottesville, VA
www.quartetbooks.com

If you are unable to order this book from your local bookseller, you may order directly from the author.
Vibrant Health
www.BCVibrantHealth.com

Library of Congress Control Number: 2015919650

ISBN 978-0-9890662-2-8
10 9 8 7 6 5 4 3 2 1

Printed on acid-free paper in the United States

*Dedicated to my brave and
loving mother, Claire V. Smith*

Contents

Norm Shealy on Whole Body Vibration

All healthy movement is good; some is superb. We were meant to move hours each day. Unfortunately, modern life has reduced by 90 percent the physical effort of day-to-day living. And although it is well proven that a *minimum* of thirty minutes of daily exercise is a basic health essential, only 10 percent of Americans get that! Just watch babies. They move a majority of the time they are awake. Fortunately, I have always felt a need to move and enjoy moving. At eighty-two years of age, I exercise a minimum of ninety minutes daily, and more on some days.

Ten years ago, after learning about what I have called vibratory exercise, I purchased a whole body vibration machine, which I use as part of my routine a minimum of five days a week. I miss it when I travel. Some days, in the late afternoon, I indulge in a second session of whole body vibration. It reenergizes me.

There are well over fifteen hundred scientific articles on the benefits of whole body vibration, including:

• improved trunk muscle strength

- improved physical function in patients with knee osteoarthritis

- improved gait speed and standing in cerebral palsied children

- improved functional exercise capacity and quality of life in those with chronic obstructive lung disease

- improved cardiac output

- decreased pain and disability in those with chronic low back pain

- better performance of distance cyclists who do WBV at their interval rest stops instead of just resting

- improved blood levels of sclerostin, critical for bone health

- improved blood sugar regulation in diabetics

- improved gait and stability in the elderly

- improved functioning in those with ADHD

Interestingly, those who need it the most benefit the most, but almost everybody will both enjoy it and benefit from doing it. Combine this with the overall energetic balancing of homeopathy, and you have a winner. For two hundred years, homeopathy has been used in the United States and around the world as the safest known alternative to drugs. Continuing scientific research makes this an ideal time to look further at the benefits of this unique and fascinating health enhancer. For those who really are couch potatoes and need movement, I urge you to read and heed the wisdom of this book. For everyone else, just enjoy adding either therapy, or both, to your health routine.

C. Norman Shealy, MD, PhD,
founder and CEO of the National Institute of Holistic Medicine,
author of *Living Bliss* and *A Physician's Encounter with Heaven*

Foreword

Burke Lennihan
on Homeopathy

In this remarkable book, Becky Chambers shares the best-kept secret in health care—homeopathy. Used worldwide by millions of people, homeopathy is virtually unknown in the US. It is part of the national healthcare system and practiced by physicians in many countries around the world, but it is dismissed by most physicians here.

Yet homeopathy has so much to offer. Powerful yet gentle, it has no side effects.* It can work almost instantaneously—as many can attest after having popped a pellet of Chamomilla into the mouth of a baby screaming with teething pain, then watching with astonishment as the baby immediately drops off into peaceful sleep. It can work for fatal diseases for which conventional medicine still has no answers: cholera,

---

*As this book explains, a homeopathic remedy can cause a temporary worsening of symptoms, called an aggravation, but this is part of the healing process and, therefore, not like the side effects caused by pharmaceutical drugs. To clarify, side effects are secondary, unintended, and undesirable toxicity effects that continue as long as the person continues to take the medication. An aggravation is a temporary increase in symptoms that can be part of the healing process. If the remedy is too strong, this aggravation can be severe and prolonged. Because of the potential for aggravations, high-potency homeopathic remedies should be used only with the help of a highly trained, professional homeopath.

plague, tuberculosis, AIDS.* It can work for common viral infections like the flu; in my own practice, clients with the flu generally bounce back in a day or two. (Most use homeopathic prevention and never get the flu at all.)

Chronic illnesses can often be resolved by addressing any underlying emotional trauma, what homeopaths call the "Never Well Since" (as in, "I've never been the same since my mother died" or "since my husband left me" or "since I lost my home in the subprime mortgage meltdown"). Part of homeopathy's healing paradigm is that unresolved emotional trauma can, in time, find an outlet through physical symptoms. It is as though the body is speaking through the language of pain what the person cannot express in words or tears. In these cases, it is only by relieving and releasing the emotional trauma that the physical condition can be healed.

Not only does homeopathy provide this insight, it provides a method of cure. A homeopathic remedy that matches the whole person —including their mental, emotional, physical, spiritual, and energetic states—can heal that person on all levels. Chronic diseases considered incurable by conventional medicine can be healed. This book provides many examples.

Homeopathy has stood the test of time. The same remedies used nearly two hundred years ago—like the ones described in this book—are still in use today. Homeopathy combines the best of East and West. It was founded by a German physician who was well schooled in the medicinal and herbal traditions of Europe, yet was inspired by the energy-healing paradigm of the East. What Traditional Chinese Medicine calls *chi* and Ayurvedic medicine calls *prana,* homeopathy calls the Vital Force.

How does it work? Homeopathy has long withstood criticisms that it can't possibly work "because there's nothing in it." Only within the past few years has conventional science developed technology powerful

---

*Homeopathy's effectiveness against these traditional scourges of humanity is part of the historical record; see Michael Emmans Dean, *The Trials of Homeopathy* (Essen, Germany: KVC Verlag, 2004). Modern homeopaths are using homeopathy to cure AIDS in Africa. See, for example, the work of Jeremy Sherr in Tanzania at http://www.homeopathyforhealthinafrica.org/.

enough to measure the minute particles of the active healing ingredient in a homeopathic remedy solution. Scientists at the Indian Institute of Technology in Mumbai (India's equivalent of MIT) recently were able to isolate these active ingredients.[1]

It turns out that homeopathy is an early form of nanopharmacology. This latest trend in conventional medicine—using tiny, barely measurable amounts of a drug to reduce its side effects and to mimic the exquisitely nanosized doses at which our hormones and other vital cell signaling agents are known to operate—was discovered two hundred years ago at the dawn of homeopathy.

How, then, do these nanodoses work? They convey both information and energy to the body's Vital Force through electromagnetic waves like the energy waves described in this book. While this may sound "woo-woo," it is not. It is at the cutting edge of physics, in particular a new branch called ultrahigh dilution physics. The electromagnetic effects of these ultrahigh dilutions were described by Nobel Laureate Dr. Luc Montagnier. In an interview with *Science* that shocked the scientific community, Montagnier asserted that his research shows how homeopathy works. He added, "The high dilutions [used in homeopathy] are right. High dilutions of something are not nothing. They are water structures which mimic the original molecules."[2]

Montagnier's research, and that of many of his colleagues, has demonstrated that the electromagnetic signals of the original medicine remain in the water of a highly dilute solution and have dramatic biological effects.

In classical homeopathy, a single remedy is given at a time, typically a high potency dose intended to last for many weeks or months. The results can be remarkable, yet the process can be slow, and it can be difficult for the patient to discern the subtle effects of the remedy on a day-to-day basis.

In this book, Becky Chambers describes a radical innovation in homeopathy—combining it with whole body vibration—to make it act much more quickly and enable clients to receive the benefits of many powerful remedies in succession. You will be inspired by her story and the stories of her clients, and you will most likely want to try high potency (very strong) homeopathy for yourself. Please do not attempt this on your own at home!

If you would like to take the material in this book one step further, read more about the fascinating personality types associated with the major remedies. My favorite books (in addition to Philip Bailey's *Homeopathic Psychology,* recommended by Becky) are Catherine Coulter's *Nature and Human Personality* and Jerry Kantor's *Toxic Relationship Cure.* In the latter book, Kantor describes remedies for people suffering from their relationship with a parent or friend, a lover, a boss, or even a religious institution.

So now you want to try homeopathy for yourself! Here are some safe ways to do it. For an acute emotional upset (you just got bad news, someone just died, you just flunked a test, or you were fired from a job), it's totally safe to use a remedy from your local health food store, such as Ignatia if you get hyperemotional with lots of sobbing and sighing or Gelsemium if you shut down and go numb. You can also use homeopathy for a wide variety of treat-at-home types of accidents and quickly passing illnesses like colds. Children love taking the little pellets, and it's very safe and effective for them.

For a long-term condition, whether physical, emotional, or both, you may identify a remedy in this book that seems to match you well. But the descriptions imbedded here within the stories are simplified to make a highly readable and enjoyable book—for the sake of good storytelling. With more than three thousand remedies from which to choose, chances are there is one even better for you than the one about which you read. That's why you need to go to a professional homeopath.*

---

*If possible, it's best to work with a professional homeopath in person. Consult the directories at www.homeopathicdirectory.com and www.nationalcenterforhomeopathy.org, and also ask around for a recommendation from your local health food store or other holistic practitioners (because the best homeopaths are often so busy, they do not list in a directory). Many communities do not have a local homeopath, however. The next best option is to find one who works using Skype. (Better yet, use an encrypted platform that protects your confidential medical information, which Skype does not. VSee is a recommended platform, at vsee.com.) Homeopaths who provide phone or video consultations are listed in the directory at www.nationalcenterforhomeopathy.org.

When you meet your professional homeopath, you will find that he or she is most likely unaware of how whole body vibration will enhance the effectiveness of her remedies. You will probably need to give her a copy of this book and ask her to consider this approach. Because it is so unfamiliar and so radically different in its time frame from the slow classical method, she will probably ask you to work with her approach first. You will still most likely get marvelous benefits from homeopathy. You can certainly point out to your homeopath the remedy that you feel matches you best, based on your reading, but you can expect that your homeopath will find an even better one that you have never heard of, so keep an open mind.

If you are doing whole body vibration at the same time, your homeopath may notice that the remedies are getting results faster, new symptom pictures are coming up faster, and you are ready for a new remedy sooner. She will follow a basic law of homeopathic healing: stay with a remedy as long as it is effective, then watch for the symptoms of a new remedy (often representing an earlier phase in the person's life).

Over time, the synergy of these two modalities will become widely known and appreciated. We may well be welcoming the dawn of a new era in energy healing, and you will be among the pioneers.

Burke Lennihan, RN, CCH,
author of *Your Natural Medicine Cabinet:*
A Practical Guide to Drug-Free Remedies for Common Ailments,
www.BurkeLennihan.com, www.YourNaturalMedicineCabinet.com

Preface

In my long journey to health, I have had to be patient as I have dealt with a seemingly endless barrage of illnesses. I have hope, though, that surmounting my latest health challenge will be the final mountain in this journey, partly because in that strange circular way of life, my latest mountain was also the first mountain.

I am a classic "canary in the mine," with an extreme sensitivity to much of modern life. When I reached adulthood more than forty years ago, my body began rebelling by developing a host of chronic physical health problems. But my story really begins with depression as a young child. This depression, at times severe, continued for thirty years. I had crippling insecurities and low self-esteem. I developed addictive eating behaviors, including bulimia, and by my early twenties, I weighed two hundred pounds. By then, I also had rampant allergies, painful digestive problems, immune system weakness, and disabling joint and nervous system maladies.

I had begun my search for health in my teens, using standard Western medicine and psychiatric care. For years there was little progress, and by my twenties the physical complaints urgently demanded attention. Out of desperation I began considering natural health, but by then so many systems in my body were involved and the situation was so complex that I had become a difficult case.

For example, I had developed early on a case of *Candida* (yeast) overgrowth. This is a gut flora disorder that in severe cases can become systemic, causing multiple symptoms and great distress. I would improve with diet changes and products or drugs to control the yeast, but within weeks I would be sick again because I had become allergic to whatever product I was taking. Because of this extreme reactivity, the doctors called me a "universal reactor." Eventually, I become allergic to more than three hundred different foods. For many years, I was able to eat only by taking daily allergy desensitization drops and rotating all foods so that no food was repeated within a five-day period.

I tried many different natural-health approaches and doctors: special diets, nutritional supplements, herbs, Chinese medicine, chiropractic care, acupuncture, heavy-metal removal by intravenous and oral chelation, allergy desensitization, and more, but I was still going downhill. By my early thirties, I could barely eat anything and had lost eighty pounds, ending up a slim 120 pounds of unhealthy, depressed, and lonely misery. My immune system was so overworked and weak that the slightest nick in my skin would lead to an infection that would take months to heal. My liver was so overwhelmed that I had developed multiple chemical sensitivities (MCS); I could eat only organic food and could not tolerate drugs of any sort.

I had been getting bladder infections twice a year for ten years when I contracted an infection that I could not eradicate. Antibiotics had always cured my bladder infections in the past, so for six months I tried three different antibiotics known to be effective against the bacteria in my bladder. Each time, I got worse, ending up with more bacteria than I started with (as determined by lab tests), along with disastrous effects on my digestive system as the *Candida* yeast would flare up wildly. I also tried several different natural approaches, all with no success.

It was at this point that I decided to try homeopathy, a form of energy medicine that I had heard about but had avoided because my background of Western science training dictated that it couldn't possibly work. My first experience with it led to a seismic shift in my thinking.

My medical doctor had said that if I did not control the bladder infection, it would travel to my kidneys, and I would soon require a kidney transplant or I would die. Under this threat, I decided to give homeopathy a shot. To my amazement, within hours of taking my first homeopathic remedy, my symptoms began to change. Within a few days, my problem was markedly better, and the infection was completely gone in one week. Remarkably, I also didn't get another bladder infection for fifteen years.

I felt that this turn of events could not be a placebo effect, because I had been sure the antibiotics would work, since they had always worked before, and I was sure the homeopathic remedy would not work. My mind opened to new possibilities.

Soon after this, I began working with Keith DeOrio, an innovative medical doctor who uses a wide range of natural approaches including homeopathy. I consulted with him monthly for many years, using and learning about homeopathy, nutritional products, specialized diets, and eventually whole body vibration—a powerful body, mind, and spirit therapy. It was all helpful, but I was especially appreciative of the homeopathy and whole body vibration; used in tandem, they are powerful in shifting a person's electromagnetic vibrational energy along with one's physical and mental health.

I went back to school and got a degree in natural health, specializing in homeopathy. By 2003, my health had improved enough that I could begin my own natural health consulting work.

When I look back at my life, I see a personal shift from one of the most miserable and least functional of people to a resilient and productive member of society. I owe much of this change to homeopathy and whole body vibration.

I have explored many avenues in my journey and have come to understand that one's energy is the key to one's health and overall well-being. Not dealing with your energy is like fighting the tide—it is an inexorable natural force. Rather than building dikes, breakwaters, and sand barriers to try to control the waters and protect your spot on the beach, if you move to higher ground, life will improve. Changing your energy helps you to change the very ground upon which you sit. It can shift your subconscious mind, changing who you think you are and enabling you to let go of the negative energy that blocks the true, bright, and shining you.

Twenty-five years after starting on this energy-tuning path, my body and mind are a well of strength and vitality. I am grateful to homeopathy because I can see what it has done for me. Let me show you how this magical yet scientific method can help you, too.

Acknowledgments

I want to thank the many homeopaths and scientists whose brilliant work, often under difficult circumstances, has paved the road for future generations. I personally have benefited, and the development of homeopathy and whole body vibration (WBV) has depended on the combined efforts of many. Particularly, I want to thank Roger Morrison, MD, Philip M. Bailey, MD, and Robin Murphy, ND, each of whom have written modern authoritative homoeopathic texts that I depend on. I especially want to thank Keith DeOrio, MD, who was my doctor and mentor for twenty years. His knowledge and innovative approaches transformed my life, and he taught me much of what I know today about homeopathy, whole body vibration, and nutrition.

I thank my clients, who, over the last fifteen years, have helped me to learn how best to use WBV to help people, particularly those clients who have allowed their stories to be told in this book. Their names and the details of their lives have been changed to protect their anonymity, but they still deserve credit for their willingness to share their personal stories. I also thank the many other clients and friends who provided valuable feedback and encouragement in the writing of this book, with special thanks to Ailie Jonston Sterry of the United Kingdom, for providing me with a European perspective; Catherine Wilkie, for her enthusiasm and storytelling instincts; and Libby Wallis, for her longtime support of my ideas and plans.

A heartfelt thanks to my family, whom I am blessed to have in my life and who have provided support, love, and safety throughout the years. My mother, Claire Smith, has my greatest respect and appreciation for her permission to use her true name in the telling of our shared story.

I thank Jeanne Mayell, MPH, for her intuitive counseling and content editing, invaluable aids in navigating the rocky shoals of the business world. Dr. Norman Shealy has provided helpful information and expertise regarding energy medicine, whole body vibration, and the brain. I thank Burke Lennihan, RN, CCH, for her support, expertise, and wonderfully open mind. Dana Ullman, MPH, is a leading proponent of homeopathy in the US. I thank him for sharing his deep and broad expertise in homeopathy.

I thank the following people for their expert professional services: editors, Tania Seymour and Ginny Weissman; interior book designer, Jane Hagaman; proofreader, Cynthia Mitchell; cover designer, Darryl Khalil; and publicist, Sara Sgarlat.

A Phoenix Rising

My Purpose

Three things cannot be long hidden:
the sun, the moon, and the truth.

—Buddha

Homeopathy and whole body vibration are forms of energy medicine, which are based in profound truths about the nature of the universe. Like the life-giving sun that is always there, shining brightly whether or not there are clouds, these energy medicine methods are a path to true healing, and they will prevail.

After searching for forty years, I have found true healing from intractable illness, using the combination of homeopathy and whole body vibration. After trying dozens of therapies, both mainstream and alternative, I found homeopathy twenty-five years ago, and I was impressed from the beginning by its power. Twelve years ago, I began adding whole body vibration to my regimen and once again saw immediate and dramatic results. As I began to understand whole body vibration, to use it properly and in conjunction with homeopathy, my healing accelerated.

While there are many books on homeopathy and several on whole body vibration, this is the first book that discusses combining the two. **While individually homeopathy and whole body vibration are valuable healing systems, together they are synergistic, igniting a healing fire of epic proportions.**

Chapter 1 introduces homeopathy, the science and history behind it, and how it is used. Chapter 2 describes whole body vibration, especially as it relates to energy medicine. Four stories of my clients using these methods follow, illustrating how the healing process works. The last chapter is my story.

Homeopathy

Often maligned and misunderstood, homeopathy actually has a long history of success. It was once so popular in the United States that along with the existence of twenty-plus homeopathic medical schools, eleven American presidents have used it, and a statue of its founder, Dr. Samuel Hahnemann, was erected in our nation's capital.

Homeopathy has been overshadowed by the rise of allopathic drug medicine since the early part of the twentieth century. During that time, the world was giddy with advancements in science and medicine. People believed that a person was cured if their symptoms could be suppressed, even though the source of the disease was still present. Allopathic, drug-oriented medicine, still dominating our medical care, did not acknowledge the interconnectivity of the body and mind as a whole organism, instead treating its parts as if they were separate.

In recent years, however, many have seen the limits of Western medicine, often tragically. There is an epidemic of chronic illness in this country that Western medicine cannot cure. Homeopathy and whole body vibration, an intensive body, mind, and spirit therapy, are growing in popularity because they cure the source of the disease and restore balance to the body and mind.

Energy medicine is the tuning of a person's vibration to a higher, more pure frequency. A lifetime of health and personal challenges has shown me that this little-known, often unaddressed phenomenon holds the key to a healthy life. This book explores the use of homeopathy, particularly when used at the same time as whole body vibration. Together they result in an accelerated and effective body, mind, and spirit therapy.

With the increasing interest in alternatives to allopathic medicine, and new discoveries in science that have begun to uncover the mystery of how homeopathy works, the time has come for a resurgence of this method of energy healing.

Whole Body Vibration

Chapter 2 introduces whole body vibration (WBV), a therapeutic system that is booming worldwide because of its remarkable capacity to enhance health and well-being (also see my website, www.BCVibrantHealth.com, and my book *Whole Body Vibration: The Future of Good Health*). WBV is intense exercise that stimulates both our muscles and our neurons to fire twenty to fifty times per second. This powerful stimulation of the nervous system causes a surge in electromagnetic energy to shoot through our body and into our brain. As energy medicine is based on electromagnetic phenomena, it is not surprising that there would be an interaction between whole body vibration and the use of homeopathy.

I will also explore cutting-edge research that links brain synchronization (the simultaneous in-phase firing of brain cells across regions of the brain) with optimal brain health, including creativity and problem solving, learning, and long-term memory formation. Whole body vibration, like a number of other therapeutic systems that stimulate the neurological system in a particular manner, may help to induce this transformative brain-wave state.

Five Stories of True Healing

The experiences of four of my clients, and my own experience, demonstrate the power of these two systems of healing. Their stories are typical of many of my clients' experiences.

Stella was being held back in life by a lack of confidence and a poor sense of self-worth. When I met her several years ago, she had recently broken up with an abusive boyfriend and was working hard but living paycheck to paycheck. By the end of her treatment, all areas of her life had shifted 180 degrees.

Betty Lou's story is a touching tale of emotional growth coupled with health improvements in several areas.

Marc suffered a brain injury in a car accident when he was only four years old. When I met him, many years later, he was hoping to reduce the medications that controlled the resulting seizures but also had debilitating side effects.

Christy is a sensitive woman holding on to pain from experiences earlier in her life. When she met Derek, sparks flew in the eternal search for true love.

The fifth case study is my own story, tracing an intensive course of homeopathy that eventually healed a looming major physical disaster before I even realized it was there. I have never heard of anybody else using homeopathy the way I have used it. Perhaps I am meant to serve as an illustration of what homeopathy and vibration can accomplish. There is also a saying that applies, "You can only go as high as you have been low."

Homeopathy and vibration help to heal the body as well as the mind. Homeopathic remedies help us let go of negative energy, which affects all aspects of life, and whole body vibration seems to accelerate the process. As a result, long-standing difficult problems suddenly improve, with noticeable change often occurring in just hours.

Chapter 1

Homeopathy

Overview

Since the practice of homeopathy began more than two centuries ago, it has been proven successful in healing the body and mind—without side effects. Homeopathic remedies use energy itself as the healing agent, a concept that has been accepted for more than four thousand years in other parts of the world and is now seeing a revival in the US.

Dr. Samuel Hahnemann was the founder of homeopathy, and his students began the first homeopathic medical school in the United States in the mid-1800s. Homeopathy gained recognition because of its success in treating the deadly epidemics of the day, including scarlet fever, typhoid, cholera, yellow fever, and pneumonia.[1]

The school's method of treatment became popular in the late nineteenth century. Numerous homeopathic medical schools were training thousands of homeopathic physicians; there were one hundred homeopathic hospitals and more than a thousand homeopathic pharmacies. Boston University School of Medicine, Hahnemann Medical School in Philadelphia, New York Medical College, University of Michigan, University of Minnesota, and the University of Iowa were among those educational institutions that had homeopathic medical schools. However, by the early twentieth century, there was a precipitous decline. By the 1920s, many of the schools had closed, and by 1950, there were barely a hundred homeopathic physicians still practicing in the United States, many nearing the age of retirement.

The decline of homeopathy's popularity was largely due to the American Medical Association's growing influence and its declaration that homeopathy was unproven medical quackery. In the late 1800s, the AMA was a poorly financed organization with little influence and low membership, but in the early 1900s, they began to align themselves with the pharmaceutical companies, promoting them in exchange for their advertising dollars. In just ten years, from 1900 to 1910, the AMA's advertising revenue increased by 500 percent, and their membership grew from eight thousand to more than seventy thousand. Their attacks on homeopathy were part of a campaign to discredit the competition in the battle for dominance in the medical world.

During that time, pharmaceutical companies began advancing drugs that were easy for doctors to administer to patients, including new painkillers that gave the illusion of a cure but had the possibility of addiction or other serious side effects. Compared to homeopathic remedies, treating patients with drugs required much less time and understanding by the physician. Allopathic medicine (still conventionally used today) and the accompanying drugs were substantially more lucrative than homeopathy, factors that also contributed to homeopathy's decline.

In contrast to using the concentrated doses of specific chemicals in drugs, homeopaths used extremely diluted doses of various plants, minerals, animals, or even chemicals chosen with great care. Rather than prescribing one medicine for everyone with the same disease as was (and is) done in conventional medicine, homeopaths individualized a specific medicine to a patient based not on simply the disease that they had, but more on the unique syndrome of symptoms of which the disease was a part. Homeopaths were capitalizing on a phenomenon in which people become hypersensitive to a substance that will cause (in a nonhomeopathic overdose) similar symptoms to those that the sick person is experiencing.

It is these extreme dilutions used in homeopathy, to the point at which—according to the current laws of physics—there should be no substantial amount of the original remedy material left, that has led to disbelief by many scientists and doctors. The latest science, however, has found that nanodoses (extremely small amounts) of the original substance remain in the dilutions—and at levels that are biologically active. There is, in fact, a new multidisciplinary field of science called hormesis devoted to the phenomenon of extremely small concentrations of substances having biological activity. I will go into more detail regarding this, and the other scientific concepts I touch on briefly here, later in this chapter.

Many people involved with homeopathy feel that the complex process of making homeopathic remedies transfers the "energy" of the original molecules to the water and that it is this energetic information that leads to healing. Today, science is beginning to support this principle. Dr. Luc Montagnier, the 2008 Nobel prize winner for his discovery of the AIDS virus, announced his support for the dilution system used in homeopathy. In a 2010 interview with *Science* magazine, he stated, **"High dilutions of something are not nothing. They are water structures which mimic the original molecules."**[2] (Emphasis mine)

In fact, there is research to indicate that each remedy substance creates its own fractal* to form snowflake-like structures of water molecules around each remedy molecule.[3] These structures are different for each starting substance and perhaps emanate the same unique original energy frequency that resonates with the person's energy.

The energetic phenomena that are theorized to underlie the effects of a homeopathic remedy are actually well accepted in Western science. Every substance is made of molecules that vibrate at a particular frequency, creating specific wavelengths of energy. If another resonating

---

*"A *fractal* is a never-ending pattern. Fractals are infinitely complex patterns that are self-similar across different scales. They are created by repeating a simple process over and over in an ongoing feedback loop" (http://fractalfoundation.org/resources/what-are-fractals/). If the replication is exactly the same at every scale, it is called a self-similar pattern.

wavelength is added, and the peaks or valleys of the two match up, they amplify each other, creating greater peaks and valleys. An example of the interaction of wavelengths can be seen with waves in the ocean—waves with coinciding peaks multiply in height, while others may pass through each other relatively unchanged.

Energy wavelengths interact in the same way, leading to dramatic effects in the physical world. An example of this phenomenon would be when a singer hits a note that causes a glass to shatter. Thus, one model of how homeopathy works is that if the correct homeopathic remedy is administered to the patient, one with resonating electromagnetic waves, the remedy will amplify the corresponding frequencies in the patient and produce results on the physical plane.

This wave resonance is thought to lead to healing because it amplifies the body's own ability to heal itself. In homeopathy, there is great respect for this ability. Symptoms are seen as the body's attempt to heal itself, as exemplified by the common symptom of a fever (now also well understood by physiologists and conventional medicine to be an important part of the body's defense against infections).

Interestingly, one sometimes experiences a brief increase in a symptom's severity after taking a homeopathic remedy, which is called an "aggravation," before the desired alleviation of that symptom and the person's overall disease. It seems likely that this brief increase could be the result of the amplification that would result from resonating waves. Many homeopaths believe that the healing that follows is connected to the release of a negative, unhealthy energy that had been stuck in the patient that is released by the homeopathic remedy.

A short-term aggravation, or "healing crisis"—that is, the temporary exacerbation of a person's symptoms before a more long-term alleviation or healing—also provides evidence that the effects of a homeopathic medicine are not a placebo response. The vast majority of people who respond to a placebo experience only the relief of symptoms, not a short-term aggravation of these symptoms before relief.

This idea of similar substances leading to healing is not new. Hippocrates, recognized as the Father of Western Medicine, as well as other notable medical figures such as Paracelsus, agreed with this principle known as the homeopathic Law of Similars, or "like cures like." In fact, the word "homeopathy" is derived from the Greek *homo*, meaning "similar," and *pathy*, "disease." This concept is the basis of conventional medicine's use of vaccines and allergy desensitization.

Typically in homeopathy, a resonating substance is found that, in its undiluted form, would cause the same symptoms that the ill person is experiencing.* In the complex process of multiple dilutions in water and shaking the mixture, the critical information is transmitted to structures that form in the water; that is, the unique snowflake-like fractals that recent research has indicated form in homeopathic dilutions.[4]

The beauty of the homeopathic method is that one can utilize, with safety, substances that would normally be toxic, because there is such a miniscule amount of the original ingredient in the final dose. This model of resonating energy would account for the dramatic results when the remedy is correct and no result at all if the remedy is not correct—if the energy resonates with the disease, then the person's immune and defense system is augmented to elicit the curative process. If the energy does not resonate, then nothing happens.

In contrast, the principle behind most allopathic medicines is to suppress the symptoms with substances that have the opposite effect on the body. For example, laxatives are used to reverse constipation, antipyretics to lower fever, antidepressants to block depression, anti-inflammatories to lower inflammation, and so on; even though the symptoms are the body's way of healing itself.

Occasionally, allopathic (modern conventional) medicine also now uses the healing effect of similar substances and sometimes substances that simply reduce a specific symptom. The word "allopathy," therefore, comes from the idea of using multiple other substances to effect a cure: *allo*, meaning "other" and *pathy* meaning "disease or suffering."

Because symptoms today are recognized as adaptations by an

---

*This principle of "like cures like" is the basis of homeopathy. Modern homeopathy has now developed additional methods for choosing homeopathic remedies, and homeopaths have seen that the remedies can have further curative effects beyond healing the similar symptoms indicated by this founding principal.

organism to defend and heal itself, using a drug that mimics that body's own defenses makes sense. While suppressing symptoms may provide immediate relief, it will not heal the underlying cause of a disease. Not allowing the body to respond to disease with symptoms may even cause a disease to go deeper into the body, resulting in more serious problems over time. Many homeopaths believe this is one of the reasons that severe, chronic physical and mental health problems are increasing in modern times. In addition, the high concentrations of toxic substances used in allopathic medicine often lead to dangerous side effects, addiction, and tolerance adaptations that require increasing amounts of the risky drugs to achieve "curative" results.

The Early Years

Dr. Hahnemann was an innovative and industrious German physician and chemist, who also translated twenty-two medical and chemistry textbooks from seven other languages into German. Combining his knowledge in different scientific fields with ideas he had found in the textbooks he was translating, he developed homeopathy, a new system of medicine. Doubting early explanations of Peruvian Bark's curative powers for malaria, he conceived the idea of testing the effect of Peruvian Bark on himself—and developed symptoms very similar to malaria.

Aware of Hippocrates's writings about finding the "simillimum" to cure a disease, Hahnemann went on to test on himself more than ninety substances, using many of the accepted medicines of the time: mercury, arsenic, belladonna, and other, more benign, substances.[5] His knowledge as a chemist led him to experimenting with different ways of preparing the substances to optimize healing while minimizing toxicity.

Allopathic medicine at that time was dependent on such methods as bloodletting, purging (vomiting), diarrhea, caustic skin agents that contained high doses of toxic substances, and other methods now considered barbaric. In contrast, Hahnemann's system was especially appealing. Popular with both the masses and the elite, it expanded rapidly throughout Europe and then to America.

In the 1800s, homeopathy particularly gained traction with its success against the deadly epidemics of the times. The recorded death rates in homeopathic hospitals during that time was typically one half to even one eighth that of conventional medical hospitals.[6, 7] Eventually, eleven US presidents, European royalty (including three generations of British royals), Russian royalty, Hawaiian royalty, and millions of people worldwide were using homeopathy with enthusiasm and success.

By the early 1900s, there were twenty-two homeopathic medical schools, one hundred homeopathic hospitals, and a corps of homeopathic medical doctors in the US armed services. President McKinley was the guest of honor at the opening ceremonies for the monument to Dr. Hahnemann in Washington, DC,[8] which then stood as the only statue of a medical doctor in our nation's capital for more than one hundred years.

Historical evidence of homeopathy's effectiveness can be seen in the death records from allopathic and homeopathic hospitals during the 1918 influenza pandemic that killed fifty million people worldwide. Homeopathic hospitals had a 1 percent death rate (treating 26,000 patients), while allopathic hospitals had a 28 percent death rate (treating 24,000) patients.[9, 10] Nearly one hundred years later, conventional medicine still has no drug that can cure the flu as quickly, as effectively, and as safely as a homeopathic remedy.

The growth of homeopathy, however, created an economic threat to allopathic doctors. Homeopathic medical doctors were claiming that allopathic medicine was doing more harm than good, criticizing especially the use of large doses of toxic substances and untested combinations of drugs. The pharmaceutical industry of the day (i.e., apothecaries) was also losing money as homeopathic medicines were, and continue to be, less profitable. Apothecaries of that time were required to charge by the amount of a substance sold, and homeopathic medicines are very dilute and time-consuming to make.

Then, as now, medicine and drugs were big business, and a threat to this industry was not taken lightly. Homeopathy was attacked as unscientific quackery, breaking the rules of science. There is a long history in science, though, of attacking new discoveries before they are accepted. Galileo, now recognized as the father of modern astronomy, first proposed that the Earth rotated around the sun but was accused of heresy and forced by the church to recant.

In the mid-1800s, the American Medical Association (AMA) was formed, partly to fight homeopathy. In the effort to discredit homeopathy, it passed rules forbidding doctors from consulting with homeopaths and eventually from even treating patients who also saw homeopaths. A physician could lose his AMA membership merely for consulting with a homeopath, hence breaking these rules was professional suicide; it meant you could lose your right to practice medicine.

As the *New York Times* editorialized in 1882, "The AMA says that if a patient's life cannot be saved except by such a consultation, then the patient must die, and no doctor who will allow a homeopathist to help him can be recognized by the Association."[11]

The discovery of new allopathic drugs and techniques in the early 1900s turned the tide against homeopathy. Impressive effects from antibiotics, aspirin, vaccinations, and X-rays made allopathic medicine easier to practice and more financially lucrative. Homeopathic medicines, on the other hand, are inexpensive and require individualized consultations that can be time-consuming.

By 1910, the AMA had produced the Flexner Report, which rated medical schools, weighting in favor of allopathic medicine. Eventually physicians could not be licensed to practice medicine if they attended a homeopathic school.[12] By 1950, there were only a hundred homeopathic physicians left in the US, and they were mostly old and near retirement.

Homeopathy in the World Today

Today the situation is vastly different. Many people have become disillusioned with an increasingly technological and expensive medical establishment dependent on drugs that are often a slippery slope. There may be initial symptomatic relief with drugs, but side effects lead to more and more pills and a decreasing quality of life. Currently, homeopathy is growing in favor in the United States, though it is still far from its former popularity.

In other parts of the world, homeopathy remains a strong and viable medical system, though it continues to encounter fierce opposition. It is widely used in Europe, Russia, India, Pakistan, and Latin America. A 2015 survey of physicians in France—a country that the World Health Organization recently listed as number one in a worldwide ranking of health care systems[13]—found that 95 percent of general practitioners, pediatricians, and dermatologists prescribe homeopathic medicines.[14]

Fifty-seven percent of people in Germany use homeopathic medicines,[15] and the German Medical Association has announced its support for homeopathy and for reimbursement for homeopathic care. In fact, it is a part of the national health care systems of quite a few countries: Germany, India, Brazil, Mexico, Pakistan, Sri Lanka, the United Kingdom, Switzerland, Italy, and France.

In India, where the status and legal position of homeopathic practitioners is similar to that of medical practitioners,[16] there are impressive numbers reported: 300,000 qualified homeopaths, 180 homeopathic medical schools, 7,500 government clinics, 307 hospitals, and 24 state boards for the registration of qualified practitioners of homeopathy.

In 2011, a book[17] was published in Switzerland (now also translated into English) that was based on a report on homeopathic medicine commissioned by the Swiss government in 2006.[18] This report represents the most comprehensive evaluation of homeopathic medicine ever undertaken by a government. The report evaluated systematic reviews and meta-analyses, outcome studies, and epidemiological research, as well as many other considerations and factors. The conclusions solidly affirmed that homeopathic treatment is both effective and cost-effective. For a brief overview of the extensive evaluations conducted, see Dana Ullman's 2013 *Huffington Post* article.[19]

An example of one such study was conducted at the University of Vienna Hospital, which found significant improvements in patients with chronic obstructive pulmonary disease (COPD),[20] a leading cause of death in the US. The amount of secretions in patients' lungs was reduced, as were their hospital stays (4.2 days instead of 7.4 days). Statistical analysis of the reduction of secretions yielded a P value of less than 0.0001, essentially meaning that the probability that these results are not true for the general population is about as likely as a person being hit by lightning sometime during their lifetime.*

For the reader looking for more detail, Dana Ullman, MPH, CCH, has authored ten books and hundreds of articles on homeopathy, making him one of the most vocal contemporary advocates on the subject. One of his eBooks references and describes more than three hundred clinical trials, published in peer-reviewed journals, testing homeopathic medicines (available at www.homeopathic.com).

People are becoming skeptical of allopathic medicines with good reason, despite the high volume of advertising that inundates us. In 2002, the ten largest drug companies in the Fortune 500 made a combined profit of $33.7 billion, more than the remaining 490 companies combined.[21] Marcia Angell, MD, a Harvard professor of medicine and former editor of the *New England Journal of Medicine*, wrote the following passage about the pharmaceutical industry:

> This industry uses its wealth and power to co-opt every institution that might stand in its way, including the U.S. Congress, the FDA, academic medical centers, and the medical profession itself.[22]

In this environment, alternative-health approaches of all types have grown to the point where, according to a government report in 2007, Americans spent $33.9 billion out-of-pocket on complementary and alternative medicine in one year.[23] Homeopathy has been growing during this period as well, but its long history of controversy and its basis in scientific principles ahead of its time have slowed its growth. Older homeopathic texts also use quaint and obscure English, which

---

*A P value of less than .0001 means there is a 1 in 10,000 chance that the results are not correct, while the chance of being hit by lightning during an eighty-year lifetime is 1 in 12,000 (https://en.wikipedia.org/wiki/Lightning_strike, as of July 2015).

can be off-putting (but the fact that two hundred-year-old texts are still in use and valid shows that homeopathy has stood the test of time). However, new research supporting the science behind homeopathy, along with a shift toward a greater appreciation of the mind-body connection, is opening the way for homeopathy to rise again.

Scientific Controversy

To understand the controversy around homeopathic medicines (also called homeopathic remedies, or just remedies), you need to know how they are made. A substance is diluted (usually 1:10 or 1:100), then shaken vigorously (called *succussion*), and the entire process is then repeated anywhere from three times to ten million times. Most remedies available in health food stores and administered by homeopaths use the 1:100 dilution method and are marked with a number (denoting the number of times the diluting and shaking process was repeated) followed by the letter C, standing for "centesimal" (referring to the hundredth dilution). The most common remedy in health food stores is 30C; this remedy and all lower numbers—such as all X (1:10 dilutions), 6C, or 12C—are considered "low potency" remedies.

The higher potencies start with 200C and go up to 1M (M is the Roman numeral for 1,000, so 1M refers to 1,000C) and beyond to 10M, 50M, and even CM, MM, and 10MM. All remedies 200C and above should be used with the guidance of an experienced professional homeopath, as these potencies can have very powerful effects on the body (that is why they are generally not sold in retail stores).

Succussion is essential to this process; just diluting a substance does not work. The whole process is called *potenizing*, because homeopaths, beginning with Dr. Hahnemann and continuing for two hundred years, have observed that the more times the process is repeated, the more powerful, or *potent*, a homeopathic remedy becomes—based on the magnitude and duration of changes in physical and mental symptoms.

Observing this phenomenon, homeopaths have theorized that the water in which remedies are diluted is changed during the process;

in fact, recent research has borne out this concept. Research showing that the structure of water can be changed by pressure applied through the process of succussion is so significant that four leading lights in the fields of material science and integrative medicine asserted: "The single argument used against homeopathy, that because there are no molecules of the remedy left in the final product it cannot be different, is completely negated."[24]

Other research has focused on identifying nanodoses of the starting materials in homeopathic dilutions. Remedies below 12C have been generally agreed (based on current understandings of physics and chemistry) to contain some molecules of the original starting substance. However, recent research has identified some of the starting molecules even in potencies above 12C, a dilution at which current laws of physics would predict none would be found.

The American Chemistry Society is not affiliated with homeopathy in any way. However, this society published in *Langmuir* (their well-respected journal) a study verifying that extreme dilutions of homeopathic drugs, made using the traditional homeopathic methodology, led to the persistence of nanodoses of each ingredient in the final solutions. Further, the nanodoses that persisted in these water solutions were at levels similar to the nanodoses at which our hormones and other vital neurological processes are known to operate.

The research published in *Langmuir* was conducted at the famed India Institute of Technology. Six different ingredients of homeopathic medicines (gold, silver, copper, tin, zinc, and platinum) were diluted 1:100 six times, thirty times, and two hundred times. Using three types of spectroscopy, the researchers found nanodoses of each of the original medicinal agents in the water solution.[25]

The new branch of science called "hormesis" has shown significant and sometimes substantial biological effects from extremely small doses of biological agents (corresponding to low potency homeopathic remedies). For example, pheromones (hormones emitted externally by animals and insects) will result in a response when as little as one molecule is received, sometimes miles from where it was emitted.[26]

Another example would be sharks in the ocean, who can sense blood miles from its source.

In humans, chemicals in the brain called beta-endorphins are known to modulate natural killer cell activity at extremely small dilutions—at levels comparable to low potency homeopathic remedies. Once disputed, hormesis is now accepted, and there have been approximately one thousand peer-reviewed studies from a range of scientific specialties confirming its validity.[27] Allopathic medicine has been taking advantage of hormesis effects for many years in vaccinations and allergy desensitization procedures.

An important concept in the field of hormesis is the idea that sensitivity is required for a reaction; that is, only an opposite sex animal or insect of the same species will react to a particular pheromone. This is true in homeopathy also; the person must have a hypersensitivity to the substance (or energy) that the homeopathic is made from for the remedy to work.

Allopathic medicine typically relies on powerful doses that will guarantee a response across a broad spectrum of people; homeopathy uses very dilute doses specific to the individual.

Returning to the idea that the water itself changes in the process of making a homeopathic remedy, Martin Chaplin, PhD, CChem, professor at South Bank University (London), studied the "memory of water." He explored the evidence for several possible mechanisms, ranging from changes in the bonds forming water molecules to the effects of silica particles found in water succussed in glass bottles. He wrote:

> There is a strange occurrence, similar to the "memory of water" but unconnected to it, in enzyme chemistry where an effectively non-existent material still has a major effect. . . . Water does store and transmit information, concerning solutes, by means of its hydrogen-bonded network. . . . Succussion may also have an effect on the hydrogen bonded network . . . with [a] critical effect on structuring.[28]

Further support comes from a group of scientists in the "material sciences," a field that integrates research from physics, chemistry, and engineering. Rustum Roy, PhD (the late head of the material sciences lab at Penn State, ranked by the Information Science Institute as the best in the world), William Tiller, PhD (the former chairman of the department of material sciences at Stanford University), Iris Bell, MD, PhD (the research director of the Program in Integrative Medicine at the University of Arizona), and M. R. Hoover, PhD (assistant professor, Materials Research Institute, Penn State) wrote an article and editorial asserting that conventional scientists have assumed that homeopathic medicines contain nothing, while ignoring that the structure of water can be changed by pressure applied through the process of succussion.[29]

Homeopaths have long believed that succussing the homeopathic remedy transfers to the water an energetic "signature" of electromagnetic waves from the original substance. It is then this energy signature that gives the remedy its biological activity. Ullman uses the analogy of a blank CD and one with music imprinted on it; they are chemically identical but carry different electromagnetic information. Further information on research regarding the science supporting and underpinning homeopathy can be found in Dana Ullman's eBook, *Evidence Based Homeopathic Family Medicine,* which can be viewed and downloaded from his website, www.homeopathic.com.

In this model, homeopathy's effects depend on resonating electromagnetic waves, which can have effects in the physical world. We are all familiar with the idea of a glass shattering when a singer hits the correct note. When a person has a resonating energy to the electromagnetic wave information contained in a homeopathic remedy, there can be a reaction.

Dr. Montagnier (the Nobel Prize winner for his discovery of the AIDS virus) supports homeopathy based on his new research investigating the electromagnetic waves that he has found emanate from the highly diluted DNA of various pathogens, diluted in the same manner as homeopathic remedies—sequential dilutions with vigorous shaking at each step. He states, "What we have found is that DNA produces structural changes in water, which persist at very high dilutions and which lead to resonant electromagnetic signals that we can measure."[30]

Dana Ullman covers this new research, and the controversy around this issue, in the *Huffington Post* online article, "Luc Montagnier, Nobel Prize Winner, Takes Homeopathy Seriously."[31] Another scientist, Dr. Jacques Benveniste, published work in *Nature* showing support for the existence of an electromagnetic memory in water of substances that were once diluted in it.[32]

Benveniste's work was vehemently denounced by the mainstream medical community, though it had been replicated in three other university laboratories, was supported by other Nobel prize–winning scientists,[33] and has been backed by further research since then.[34] Montagnier, reports Ullman in his *Huffington Post* blog, considers Benveniste to have been "attacked for investigating a medical and scientific subject that orthodoxy had mistakenly overlooked and even demonized."[35]

Choosing the Correct Remedy

Homeopathic remedies are chosen based on a total symptom picture, including mental and physical symptoms. It was noticing the correlation of symptoms between Peruvian Bark and malaria that first led to Dr. Hahnemann's discovery and development of homeopathy. His results and those of many other homeopaths and volunteers during the last two centuries, testing hundreds of substances, have yielded vast stores of clinical information in homeopathic texts. Homeopaths use this information along with patient interviews to determine the correct remedy.

In choosing a remedy, the patient's mental state has long been recognized to be of critical importance. Hahnemann devoted a chapter to this—"The Mental and Emotional State: Chief Ingredient of All Diseases"—in his *Organon of the Medical Art*. In it he states that there is always a mental/emotional component to chronic diseases.[36] (Hahnemann, an early pioneer in the field of public health, recognized that many diseases are also caused by lifestyle factors, such as eating a poor diet or living in a damp and moldy basement, but they may still be influenced by the mental/emotional state.)

I have found homeopathy to be a mind-opening opportunity to experience firsthand the connections between the mind, electromagnetic energy, and the physical world. A remedy is often selected with the patient's mental state as a primary consideration (which is why I will be delving into these issues in the five stories of healing in later chapters).* The physical symptoms are important when choosing a remedy, but for the homeopathic remedy to succeed in alleviating the physical symptoms, homeopaths have found that it should also match on the level of the mental state.

When both conditions are met, and a remedy is found that truly resonates with the person's energy, then both the mental/emotional state and the physical state will change, often rapidly and dramatically. Many homeopaths find that high potency remedies are needed for significant lasting change at the mental and emotional levels. However, particularly for highly sensitive individuals, low potency remedies may also alleviate emotional distress.

In the case of a high potency remedy, where the homeopathic is so diluted that it contains only energetic information, this becomes a powerful demonstration that "energy" is a force that can change the physical world and that our energy is linked to our thoughts.†

Theoretically, of course, these connections are always there, but for the average person it is a difficult thing to accept. In the case of the correct homeopathic remedy, the effect of energy on the physical world and its connection to our minds becomes clearer, and there is nothing like a personal experience to make an impression.

When the correct remedy is found, it must also be given at the

---

*There are quite a few different schools of thought on how to prescribe homeopathic medicines. This method of focusing on the emotional and mental state, and often using higher potencies, is the method that I primarily use, but success in alleviating symptoms can be achieved with different methods.

†There is now some evidence that all homeopathic medicines may have crude (molecular) doses of the original medicinal agent, even in the highest potencies. However, there are also certain styles of practicing nontraditional homeopathy in which only the *energy* of an original substance is used in the preparation of the homeopathic medicine, and these methods also appear to be successful.

proper potency to achieve a positive effect. Low potency homeopathics, such as 6C, are typically used when a person has a relatively minor acute ailment, is frail, or their vitality is low. The most common potency in health food stores is 30C, and it is suitable for home prescribing for both physical and emotional acute (short-term) conditions. High potency remedies are more powerful and are often used by homeopaths for chronic conditions, both physical and mental/emotional.

The strength of the remedy, or *potency,* is important and depends on the individual situation. Too high a potency of the correct remedy could lead to a prolonged worsening of symptoms. **The potential for aggravations is an important reason why you should only use high potency remedies with a well-trained and experienced homeopath. This is also the reason why high potency remedies are not sold in retail stores.**

Many homeopaths, especially in the past, believed that only one remedy should be needed—that if you could find the true "simillimum," that would cure all symptoms. In modern times, most homeopaths recognize that there may be layers of pathology and that each layer requires a different remedy. One may even need to go through successive potencies of one homeopathic, increasing the potency gradually so as to strengthen the person enough to tolerate a higher potency dose.

Philip M. Bailey, a well-known homeopath worldwide, describes his approach using high potency remedies to address psychological issues:

> In my experience, the 10M potency [this is a high potency remedy of 10,000 dilutions] is the most effective in bringing about lasting psychological improvement, and I give it in most cases of psychological pathology unless the body is too frail to take it, or there is a danger of serious physical aggravation. In these cases the potency can be raised stepwise over several months, strengthening the body to the point where it can take higher potencies safely. . . . Considerable aggravations do occur when the potency has not been raised

stepwise, and the patient should be warned of these, assured that they are part of the process of healing, and will be followed by great psychological improvement.[37]

In this passage, Bailey refers to the phenomenon of "aggravations," where you first briefly worsen before improving. This is common with high potency homeopathics because they are so powerful. A similar phenomenon is also seen and recognized in allopathic medicine and other types of natural health. A "Herxheimer's reaction" is a term used in allopathic medicine to describe symptoms that initially increase as toxins are release when an infectious organism is killed off by drugs or another method. The term "healing crisis" is also used to describe this type of phenomenon, applying, for example, to Herxheimer's reactions and/or initially feeling ill due to the release of toxins during detoxification, such as can happen from a sauna, massage, or herbal and nutritional supplements that cause detoxification.

Aggravations may be a result of the amplification of energy that would be the result of the conjunction of resonating energy waves. As that energy is causing the symptoms in the first place, those symptoms may suddenly increase as that energy increases in the process of letting go. Aggravations can be uncomfortable and even scary, as the very symptom that you are worried about suddenly gets worse, but I am encouraged when I encounter these reactions. Aggravations confirm that you have chosen the correct remedy, that there is indeed a resonance with this energy, and that you will soon be better. Low potency remedies, on the other hand, are gentle and generally do not cause aggravations. For this reason, they are sold at retail stores and are safe for people to try on their own.

One reason I like the analogy for homeopathy of a singer hitting a note and a glass shattering is because it illustrates the dramatic nature of the reaction that can happen. I also like this analogy because the rigid but fragile nature of glass reflects the rigid, brittle nature of our psychic defenses, our stuck energy. Another point is that once that energy is broken, it will drift away with little to no effort on our part, as the water inside a broken glass would release and eventually evaporate. Evaporation takes time, but high potency homeopathics also take time to achieve their full effect (usually six to twelve months). The four stories of my clients serve to illustrate both the short- and long-term effects of homeopathy.

The science fiction writer H. G. Wells, another believer in the power of ideas and the truth, once wrote, "Kings and empires die; great ideas, once they are born, can never die . . ."[38] The phoenix represents immortality and the ability in each of us to rise up stronger and wiser from illness and defeat. Homeopathy can help us in our quests for health and happiness; and it is itself a phoenix, once crushed and hidden in the ashes of war but full of power, now rising again stronger and more beautiful than ever.

Chapter 2

Whole Body Vibration

Overview

Whole body vibration (WBV) is a therapeutic system that forty years' worth of research has documented as an intensive exercise system that has many benefits for the body, mind, and spirit (see my website, www.BCVibrantHealth.com, and my book *Whole Body Vibration: The Future of Good Health*). In this book, I will focus on its effects on our neurological and energetic systems. These effects are so powerful that very little vibration is needed to produce large results—I often see major changes after just a few minutes of gentle vibration. I have also observed to be true an idea that Dr. Keith DeOrio first proposed: using WBV in conjunction with homeopathy accelerates and augments the benefits of homeopathic treatment.

When you stand on a vibration plate, you can feel the vibration going through your body as a sensation similar to a massage. It seems simple, but every cell and molecule in your body vibrates, leading to a cascade of effects throughout your body and every aspect of your being.

On the physical level, vibration causes all of your muscle fibers to involuntarily activate so that they tighten and relax at the same speed at which the plate is vibrating, twenty to fifty times per second. That effect, plus the increase in gravity as your muscles hold your weight against vibration, leads to the beneficial results.

Ten minutes of WBV equals one hour of conventional weight lifting, leading to increased muscle strength, bone density, flexibility, coordination, balance, and weight loss. Hard to believe, but for a quick visual image, picture a man using a jack hammer and the arm and shoulder muscle development that results. WBV is much gentler and more enjoyable than this comparison, but the idea is similar. For example, if you are in a squatting position on a vibration plate, your leg muscles have to hold your body weight against the vibration, and if you are using a powerful vibration machine, that is not easy!

Exercise has been shown to be the most important factor for brain health, stimulating neural cell growth and strength. WBV is exercise on steroids. When you are on a vibration plate, all of your neurons are shooting signals to your brain, and through all the neurons in your body, twenty to fifty times per second—a massive neurological stimulation. Just as your muscles grow stronger with use, so does your brain and entire neurological system.

The big increase in electromagnetic signals shooting around your body from direct stimulation of neurons and through other less obvious effects (that I will go into later in this chapter) seems to result in an increase in the strength of this electromagnetic, or chi, energy and of its rate of change—that is, buried negative energy rises to the surface more quickly.

In natural health, it is often thought that negative energy and its associated physical and mental symptoms are stored in our bodies and minds like the layers of an onion. In other words, energetic disturbances accumulate, one on top of the other, in the order that they occur. When letting go of negative energy, you release that energy that is at the surface, which then allows an earlier energetic disturbance to rise to the surface, where it too can then be released. But you can only release a negative energy that has come to the surface; you must release the top layer first, then wait for the next layer to rise to the surface.

Before I began using WBV, under the guidance of Dr. DeOrio, I took an average of three to five high potency homeopathic remedies per year for fifteen years. After I began vibrating, that number increased to ten to fifteen per year. I have also seen this same pattern with many of my own clients over the last fifteen years. How much homeopathy a person needs will also depend on their health, of course. Some people have less severe problems than others and have correspondingly fewer negative energy layers.

One might think that WBV was causing health problems and therefore more homeopathics were needed to deal with these symptoms, but that is not the case. I see, both in myself and with my clients, an overall increase in physical and mental health and strength, leading to corresponding increases in our abilities and achievements in life. We seem to be growing and developing as human beings, sparks of light and energy with all the complexity and potential that implies, at a faster rate.

Dr. DeOrio believes that whole body vibration ramps up our energetic system, similar to WBV's effects on our metabolic system. WBV is intense exercise that stimulates both our muscles and our neurons to fire twenty to fifty times per second. Like any exercise, this causes an increase in metabolism, but this powerful stimulation of the nervous system and our electromagnetic energy seems to cause a ramping up of these systems also, leading to rapid changes there as well.

Detoxification is another area where there may be parallels between the physical and energetic effects of WBV. When vibrating muscle fibers contract around lymphatic vessels, one of the body's primary natural detoxing systems, they force the lymph to move. The lymph carries toxins and waste products from our cells out of our bodies. In addition, WBV causes increased circulation of the blood, which brings more nutrients and oxygen to all the cells, helping them to function at a higher level and therefore dump more toxins and waste products into the lymphatic system.

Perhaps by increasing the electromagnetic energy in our system with WBV we are causing these buried negative energies to rise to the surface more rapidly. And strengthening our energy allows us to tolerate the stress of releasing negative energy that can sometime result from aggravation reactions.

Brain and Nervous System

Whole body vibration can be life changing in its effects on the nervous system and brain. Immediate effects include rapidly rising levels of two neurotransmitters, serotonin and norepinephrine, that have positive effects on mood and energy levels. Serotonin is a neurotransmitter in your brain that contributes to sounder sleep and feelings of mastery, pleasure, and relaxation. This is the same neurotransmitter that is targeted by prescription antidepressant drugs such as Prozac and Wellbutrin, as well as many street drugs such as marijuana, cocaine, and Ecstasy.

While prescription drugs for depression can be valuable for helping to alleviate symptoms, they also have side effects, and they can lead to increasing tolerance of and dependence on those drugs. Whole body vibration is a natural, safe, rapid, nonaddictive, and legal way to increase serotonin and norepinephrine.

Norepinephrine is both a neurotransmitter and a hormone, and low levels of this essential molecule have been linked to depression and low energy. Norepinephrine (along with epinephrine) underlies the fight-or-flight response, giving the body sudden energy in times of stress. It increases the heart rate, triggers the release of glucose from energy stores, increases blood flow to skeletal muscles and oxygen supply to the brain, and can suppress nerve inflammation.

Studies done on rats have shown rapid increases in serotonin levels with WBV,[1] but physical measurements of brain serotonin levels can only be done in animals (as brain tissue samples must be taken). Anecdotal evidence of increased serotonin and norepinephrine levels with WBV in humans is strong. Hundreds of my clients, and many thousands of users around the world, report rapid and dramatic improvements in mood, energy, and sleep within days of beginning vibration. As of the end of 2015, Googling "whole body vibration improves mood" resulted in 232,000 hits. My clients also report increased motivation, focus, and activity levels. This is an area of great potential and should be investigated more thoroughly.

In addition, exercise has been shown to be the most important factor for brain health, leading to increased neural cell growth and strength. In fact, the latest research is that nothing helps your brain develop and stay healthy more than exercise. A recent *New York Times* magazine article, "Jogging Your Brain," states, "For more than a decade, neuroscientists and physiologists have been gathering evidence of the beneficial relationship between exercise and brainpower. But the newest findings make it clear that this isn't just a relationship; it is *the* relationship. . . . Exercise, the latest neuroscience suggests, does more to bolster thinking than thinking does."[2]

Neurogenesis is the creation of new neurons in the brain and throughout the body. This was once thought to happen only before birth, but it is now known that, at a slower pace, neurogenesis in at least the brain does continue throughout life. Neurogenesis allows for brain "plasticity," meaning that the brain can continue to grow and change throughout life, making new neural connections that allow you to not only learn new skills and knowledge but also to increase your ability to learn, think creatively, and change.

Reports of neurogenesis in the peripheral nervous system are rare, but I have had numerous clients with peripheral neuropathy (pain, numbness, loss of function) who saw dramatic improvements with WBV. I suspect that the intense stimulation of WBV is leading to growth and health in the peripheral nervous system as well as in the brain.

Research showing this connection between exercise and the brain has primarily been done with aerobic exercise. However, similar neurological and muscular processes are involved with weightlifting-type exercises, to which WBV is most similar. Perhaps WBV, with its massive neurological stimulation, will eventually be found to stimulate brain development even more effectively than other forms of exercise; scientific research in this area is eagerly awaited.

Electromagnetic Chi Energy

Whole body vibration has powerful effects on our electromagnetic, or chi, energy. Every time you are on a vibration plate, all your neurons are activated, shooting electromagnetic energy through your body and brain; and this electromagnetic energy is fundamentally connected to our physical and mental states. The electromagnetic nature of our brains is recognized by modern allopathic medicine; electroencephalography (EEG) measures electronic brain waves, and magnetic resonance imaging (MRI) creates images of the brain by measuring its electromagnetic energy.

On an even deeper level, quantum physics describes the world of subatomic particles that makes up all matter and from which electromagnetic energy arises. Quantum physicist Ervin Lazlo explains that science is in the midst of a "shift from matter to energy as the primary reality. . . . There is no categorical divide between the physical world, the living world, and the world of mind and consciousness."[3] Norman Shealy, MD, PhD, describes this connection: "A quantum universe is a set of probabilities, susceptible to influence by many factors, including thought, will, and intention."[4]

Many cultures throughout time have recognized the existence of a life-force energy. The Chinese call it chi, Indians call it prana, and European traditions have called it variously life force, soul, spirit, vital energy, vital principle, elan, and more. This energy guides and powers one's body and life, and disturbances in this energy due to trauma of any sort can have a profound effect on your physical and mental state.

Thousands of years ago, the Chinese discovered and mapped "energy meridians" in the body. Each of these energy pathways is associated with different organs and bodily systems. The Chinese medical system of acupuncture is based on maintaining a healthy and balanced flow of energy between those different meridians.

Ayurvedic medicine (developed thousands of years ago in India and still in use today) describes chakras, spinning energy vortexes in our bodies, that are also associated with particular body systems and organs. In fact, some people can sense their own vibrational energy, and when these people stand on a vibrating plate, they report feeling energy shooting through their energy meridians—and their chakras unblocking and spinning faster.

There is, in fact, measurable electromagnetic energy emanating from all things. This is because all substances are made from molecules that are, in turn, made from even smaller vibrating particles that have positive or negative electrical charges. Thus, every substance has an electromagnetic charge that can be measured with sensitive scientific equipment. For example, Kirlian photography can detect and record the electromagnetic wavelengths around a person or object.[5]

Piezoelectricity

In addition to causing our neurons to fire, WBV stimulates electromagnetic energy through a physical property of crystals called *piezoelectricity*—the ability of crystals to turn mechanical vibration into electrical vibration. Our bodies are living liquid crystals in the sense that we are highly organized molecular structures, and as such we have the property of piezoelectricity.

Dr. Shealy describes our "bodies, souls, minds, and emotional realm" as "a living matrix" with the property of piezoelectricity.[6] "Waves of mechanical vibration moving through the living matrix produce electrical fields and vice versa. . . . Connective tissue is a liquid crystalline semiconductor. Piezoelectric signals from the cells can travel throughout the body in this medium."[7] The result is that "energetic treatment of one part of this living matrix always affects the whole."[8]

Thus, every time you are on a vibration plate, your neurons fire, shooting electromagnetic energy through your body and brain; then your body turns the mechanical vibration into the electrical energy vibrations you need to heal, balance, and unblock your energy system. Energy flows into and through your energy meridians and chakra energy centers, increasing their proper spinning and energy flow. Since these energy meridians and chakras are linked to different organs, body systems, emotions, and needs, improving the flow of energy helps heal the physical body and mind and improve life—all at the same time.

Brain Synchronization—a Missing Link?

Brain synchronization is the simultaneous, in-phase firing of brain cells across regions of the brain. These combined signals generate electromagnetic brain waves, which can be measured by electroencephalography (EEG) and magnetic resonance imaging (MRI). Cutting-edge research has linked the phenomena of brain synchronization to optimal brain function and health, including creativity, problem solving, learning, and long-term memory formation. The opposite state, one of asynchronous brain wave activity, has been linked to disease states such as ADD, schizophrenia, depression, traumatic brain injury, and others. Synchronized brain waves seem to foster the formation of new synaptic connections, or brain plasticity and learning.*

Earl Miller, the Picower Professor of Neuroscience at MIT and the senior author of a study published in *Neuron* in June 2014, has been studying the effects of brain synchronization. According to Dr. Miller in an interview with the MIT news office, he has found that "the phenomenon of brain-wave synchronization likely precedes the changes in synapses, or connections between neurons, believed to underlie learning and long-term memory formation."[9]

Brain plasticity (the formation of new connections between brain cells) has been known for some time now to be a critical element for learning. However, brain plasticity, meaning the actual growth of neurons, takes too long to account for the human mind's flexibility. How the brain can process and utilize new information almost instantly has remained a mystery. As Miller explains, "Plasticity doesn't happen on that kind of time scale. The human mind can rapidly absorb and analyze new information as it flits from thought to thought. These

---

*There have been many studies to back these claims. Please see the "Brain Synchronization" section under Additional References at the back of the book.

quickly changing brain states may be encoded by synchronization of brain waves across different brain regions."[10]

Miller further describes the link between brain-wave resonance and brain development with an intriguing allusion to separate voices joining together; that is, waves of sounds: "There is some unknown mechanism that allows these resonance patterns to form, and these circuits start humming together. That humming may then foster subsequent long-term plasticity changes in the brain, so real anatomical circuits can form. But the first thing that happens is they start humming together."[11]

Synchronized wavelengths from an outside source can cause "brain entrainment," the synchronization of brain waves. This has been studied with sound and light, and linked to increases in creativity, memory, learning, problem solving, and intuition, as well as to improvements in depression, anxiety, and ADHD. Biofeedback, which can be used to treat mental health issues, also takes advantage of brain entrainment. There are now numerous companies promoting sound entrainment CDs for better brain function.

Whole body vibration has profound effects on our neurological systems. Certain types of whole body vibration deliver a completely synchronized message into the nervous system, which might lead to brain entrainment. I believe this would be a fertile area for research, having seen great benefits and changes in mental health in both my clients and myself with whole body vibration.

There are currently differences of opinion on how different types of vibration effect our bodies and nervous systems. It is theoretical at this point, but Dr. DeOrio, for example, feels that there is a risk that oscillation systems may also cause desynchronization, particularly, perhaps, in more sensitive people.[12] I would also like to see more research exploring the effects of different types of vibration on brain synchronization and on other aspects of our bodies and nervous systems.

WBV has an unprecedented ability to work on the physical, mental, and energetic levels all at once. The powerful effects on our neurological and electromagnetic systems may be why energy changes and homeopathic use often increase when using WBV. However, the very power that WBV has to affect our bodies, minds, and spirits is what makes it so important to use it correctly. One could compare WBV to fire—it has the power to change the world, but if you don't use it properly, it can also burn your house down.

My Experience with Brain Desynchronization

To achieve greater power, thus a greater workout effect, many WBV machines have two motors in them. However, as any engineer can attest, it is impossible to ever completely synchronize two motors. This lack of complete synchronization in the message sent through your nervous system and energy field by double-motor machines will have a desynchronizing effect on your nervous system and energy field, which can have negative consequences over time. While people cannot detect the millisecond lack of synchronization on a conscious level while on a WBV machine, your nervous system and energy fields are extremely sensitive, and, on a deeper, unconscious level, they will be picking up this message.

Health effects from this desynchronization can be difficult to recognize and detect. Since the athletes typically using this type of machine have such strong overall health, this subtle side effect may go unnoticed for years. By the time trouble begins to develop (and since it involves the nervous system and energy fields, it can show up as any type of problem), these users have seen so many positive effects that they do not suspect they may be using the wrong sort of vibration machine.

For me, as the sensitive canary in the mine, problems quickly become dramatic and clear. After my first year with one of these double-motor machines, during which I did see improvements and became stronger than I had been in many years, my health suddenly deteriorated. I experienced a sudden and mysterious downturn and had such severe muscle weakness that I could not make it up the stairs or even across the room (this after climbing Mt. Washington only two weeks earlier), and my allergies, chemical sensitivities, multiple infections, digestive distress, and nervous-system problems all returned. It seemed to be linked to the vibration somehow, as I would get much worse after the slightest amount, but what exactly about the vibration was bothering me was difficult to determine.

Dr. DeOrio, who I was working with at the time, theorized that it was a desynchronization effect from the double-motor machine that was causing my sudden downturn. After much trial and error, it became clear that he was correct; only desynchronizing vibration was causing problems, not single-motor vertical vibration, which provides a fully synchronized signal to one's nervous system and chi energy. In fact, I only fully recovered by using a single-motor vertical vibration system. I have now been exclusively using single-motor vertical vibration machines for eight years without a problem. The always perfectly synchronized message from these machines helps your neurological and energetic systems to synchronize themselves while still providing all the other benefits of vibration.

Thus, because double-motor machines can cause brain desynchronization, and because of my personal experience, I recommend only single-motor, vertical (also called linear) vibration. Whole body vibration has many wonderful benefits, but the issue of brain synchronization and optimal brain functioning in general is critical to long-term benefits and health. See my website, www.BCVibrantHealth.com, and book, *Whole Body Vibration: The Future of Good Health,* for more information.

NOTE: All homeopathics used in the following five stories (chapters 3–7) are high potency homeopathic remedies unless otherwise noted. Sometimes, I start people at a low potency and build up further as needed. Other times, depending on the person and the situation, I might use a higher potency remedy right from the beginning. However, for simplicity and smoother storytelling, I have not specified the exact potency level for each remedy in the stories.

High potency remedies are more powerful and are often used by homeopaths for chronic conditions, both physical and mental/ emotional. High potency homeopathic remedies should be used only with the guidance of a highly trained professional homeopath because of the potential for severe "aggravation" reactions. See "Choosing the Correct Remedy" in chapter 1 for more information on when and how high and low potency homeopathic remedies are used.

Chapter 3

Stella

Stella is a talented and empathetic thirty-eight-year-old beautician. She first came to me four years ago for whole body vibration, having heard that it could give you energy, improve your mood, help you to lose weight, and tone your muscles—all at the same time. Stella was chronically tired, not sleeping well, and, like many of us, struggling to stay in shape in the midst of a busy life. She started out with vibration sessions twice a week and saw great results almost immediately. Her mood improved, her energy level jumped, and she was losing inches and gaining strength rapidly. Stella was hooked and began to come regularly.

As I got to know Stella, it turned out that she was struggling more than she initially had let on. She had been in a serious relationship several years earlier that had ended tragically, and since then, she'd had a painful history of codependent, unhealthy relationships with men, ranging from disastrous to mediocre. She had yet to truly recover from the accidental sudden death of her fiancé four years earlier and had been on antidepressant medications for years.

Traumatized and in shock, Stella had ended up in another relationship shortly after her fiancé's death, but this rebound relationship was a disaster. He turned out to be a drug addict who was physically and emotionally abusive, and he racked up heavy debt on her credit cards (which dogged her for years afterward). When this relationship finally ended several years later, she had moved on to a relationship that was not overtly abusive, but it was unsatisfying and going nowhere. This is where she was, and had been for several years, when I met her.

Stella was also stuck in her career. She is a talented beautician, but she was not reaping the financial rewards she deserved. She had spent many years working in well-known beauty salons, and for years had wanted to open her own salon, but she lacked self-confidence, and, so far, the problems involved with striking out on her own had been too daunting.

Stella's health was reasonably strong, but there were a few stubborn issues she had been dealing with for many years that just would not go away. Like most of us, she was perennially struggling to stay in shape and not gain weight; in addition to being on antidepressant medications, she had trouble sleeping and was chronically tired. It was at this point, about six months after she first started working with me, that I began giving Stella homeopathics in addition to whole body vibration.

The first homeopathic I gave Stella was for the sadness and grief from her fiancé's sudden death, still unresolved and lingering, though hidden under her hard-working, responsible exterior. Natrum Muriaticum is a major grief remedy particularly associated with "depression, . . . silent grief," and "closed, responsible, dignified" people "much affected by grief" who are "easily offended or wounded."[1]

When I first met Stella, this description fit her, though it no longer does. After a few days of increased depression, part of the common and expected initial aggravation reaction with high potency homeopathics, Stella's mood improved, and she felt stronger emotionally than she had in a long time. Shortly after taking this remedy, Stella stopped taking her antidepressant medications, and she has never gone back to them.

A couple of months after that, I gave Stella a dose of Thuja, a classic remedy for depression, low self-esteem, and feelings of worthlessness in a person who "feels unattractive or spends much time perfecting the appearance."[2] After the initial week, during which she felt worse than ever during the aggravation period, she was suddenly stronger and more assertive. Stella was still pleasant with her clients, but she was not being walked on anymore.

Stella told me about one particularly difficult woman who had been "torturing" her for years. This time when she began complaining, Stella told her, "There are lots of other hair stylists in the salon, and I would be happy to match you up with someone else who could make you happier." And that is what happened, but not long after, this hard-to-please client was back with Stella, now treating her with respect and consideration.

This episode made a big impression on Stella, convincing her that the homeopathic remedies really were doing something, as she had been getting walked on for years and had never before been able to find the right way to handle these situations. Stella was also becoming more assertive in her romantic relationship, but her boyfriend was set in his ways, so there was little change in the situation.

A couple of months after this, Stella suddenly developed intense nerve pain in one of her legs, so severe that even on narcotic pain killers she could not sleep. I gave her Argentum Metallicum, for "electric shock sensations, especially in sleep or on going to sleep," where the "pain and symptoms appear suddenly," accompanied by an "extroverted and cheerful" personality with "impulsiveness, suggestibility, and fearfulness . . . often pathologically open."[3] This was a good description of Stella, and her situation, at that time.

She took this remedy every day for one month, and, for the first couple of weeks, the pain would disappear entirely shortly after taking the remedy, then begin to come back a few hours before she took the next dose. Gradually, the pain tapered off entirely until, by the end of the month, she no longer needed the remedy at all.

At this point, now several months after the first Thuja dose for depression and feelings of worthlessness and unattractiveness, this issue had come back. Another layer of this negative energy had surfaced, a common occurrence in the process of letting go of a negative energy. I gave Stella another, higher potency dose. Shortly after this second dose of Thuja, which released this negative "worthlessness" energy that was at the root of what had kept her shackled in a relationship that only confirmed and reinforced these feelings, she broke up with her uncommitted and unmotivated boyfriend. This turned out to be just the first of quite a few break-ups with the guy, but it was the beginning of a permanent split.

A few months later, Stella was in a minor car accident. She was not hurt beyond a few bumps and bruises; however, the accident did kick up the post-traumatic stress disorder (PTSD) she had developed from her years with the earlier abusive, drug addicted boyfriend. I gave her a remedy called Aconite, which is used when "complaints begin after a fright or sudden, shocking event."[4] Aconite can be used to counteract sudden shocks causing a fear of death, one manifestation of PTSD. Within a couple of days of beginning Aconite, Stella's restlessness was gone, and her high stress, on-alert state was calming down.

Stella was discouraged about her relationship (still going nowhere) and about her work situation. She was working hard but was dependent on bosses and coworkers who weren't as committed and conscientious as she was. Under this stress, Stella eventually slid back into depression and a constant state of exhaustion.

This time I gave her Phosphoricum Acidum, a classic remedy for chronic fatigue; especially for "depressed apathetic patients . . . ailments from grief or disappointed love . . . collapse states from grief, illness, drug, or alcohol abuse."[5] Stella took this remedy daily for two months, gaining strength and stamina until she was able to maintain her energy without needing the remedy.

Stella had become emotionally stronger and generally more cheerful, but there was still a side of her that was insecure. Her fear of rejection was holding her back in life, dampening her true bright and optimistic nature. And now her knees and wrists had begun to bother her, limiting her life and activities. Her doctor diagnosed her wrist pain as carpal tunnel syndrome, and she had begun wearing wrist braces.

This time I gave her Rhus Toxicodendron, for "cheerful, joking, and very lively" people who are "quick witted and friendly yet peculiarly timid."[6] Rhus Tox is also famous for its effects on the joints, especially for arthritis. Within a few days of starting this remedy, her joints were no longer bothering her, and she was dancing up a storm in the evening, exercising at the gym, and able to work comfortably again without the wrist braces.

All was well for several months, then Stella's allergies, which had never been severe in the past, suddenly flared up. In the mental realm, Stella's money worries had come to the fore again. She was still in debt, and business was slow, so her income was down. She was so anxious that she was having trouble sleeping, and she would sometimes have panic attacks in the middle of the night.

I gave Stella a high potency dose of Arsenicum, a classic remedy for anxiety with "panic attacks, especially after midnight," in a "proper, tense, and worried person" with fears about health and poverty (along with many other possible fears).[7] Arsenicum is also associated with depression, a need for control, perfectionism, and, on the physical level, allergies—all of which described Stella well at this time.

At the high potency level, Stella's allergies and sleep improved, and, theoretically, we could hope that her financial state would improve, too. It can take up to six to twelve months, though, to see the full effect of a high potency homeopathic.

A few more months went by, during which I frequently heard about Stella's boyfriend troubles. The situation with him was never great, and there were often fights during which it looked like the relationship would be over, but they always made up and got back together again, starting the cycle over. Stella could not get herself to leave the relationship, though the situation was driving her crazy.

I gave Stella Calcarea Phosphoricum, a remedy particularly suited to a bright and bubbly personality who is determined to hold onto the safety of "home"—that which is familiar. Calcarea is made from the shells of oysters, animals that anchor themselves to rocks and never leave—thus all Calcarea remedies (there are several versions) have the hallmark characteristic of "inertia"—a difficulty in letting go of what seems like the safety of home.[8] Phosphoricum people are bright and bubbly, so this combination remedy suited Stella. In addition, the person in the Calc Phos state is likely to be "peevish and discontented . . . complaining, never satisfied,"[9] exactly describing Stella's behavior and mental state over the last month or two.

On the physical level, this remedy is associated with a person who puts on weight quickly and easily and craves sweets. Stella and I had also been regularly commiserating on the impossibility of staying in shape through a New England winter, during which you can't exercise or be outside for long periods of time; you are stuck inside, next to all the tempting goodies. Stella's neck had also been very stiff, a typical Calc Phos symptom.

I gave her three doses of Calc Phos over three weeks. About a week after the third dose, Stella broke free with ease from her four-year relationship, splitting up for the last time with her going-nowhere boyfriend. Stella was surprised at how well she survived the break up. She was not upset, unlike all the other times she had broken up with him only to get back together shortly thereafter. She felt sure she had done the right thing and had no regrets. Calc Phos changed her energy, allowing her to more easily let go of the illusion of safety that her long-term relationship had been giving her.

Stella did become exhausted again a few weeks after the breakup, and she developed a urinary tract infection. I gave her Equisitum, well known for its actions on the kidneys and bladder. Stella had lost "Kidney Fire" because of losing someone she was close to. "Kidney Fire" is the Chinese term for chi—one's life force or electromagnetic energy—reflecting the Chinese belief that this energy originates and is centered in the kidneys. The loss of Kidney Fire left Stella's associated urinary tract vulnerable, resulting in a bladder infection. Within a few days of starting the Equisitum, her symptoms were gone.

Despite Stella's cheerful exterior, there was an element of grief from this recent relationship breakup lurking below the surface. Soon she needed Naturum Carbonicum, for "gentle, refined, selfless people . . . sadness and grief" that is hidden under a "cheerful demeanor, excessively cheerful."[10] On the physical level, this remedy matched her increased digestive troubles, her stomach having become upset after a late-night encounter with chocolate—"dyspepsia; indigestion; weak digestion, worse dietary indiscretions."[11]

All was well for several months. Stella was focused on her work and her dream of opening her own salon. Though she was anxious about money issues, as the summer ended, she made the big move, leaving her secure job and opening her own beauty salon. It was a scary leap, and her anxiety level skyrocketed. How would she manage to pay all her bills, and what would happen if she failed? Stella went into overdrive trying to control her situation, compulsively checking numbers, orders, and cleaning the shop premises; and, again, she could not sleep.

Arsenicum characteristics, along with the hallmark high anxiety, include "a need for control, perfectionism, fastidiousness," and insomnia.[12] When the same symptom picture returns after initially disappearing, it can mean that a deeper layer of that negative energy has risen to the surface. I gave Stella another dose of Arsenicum, one potency level up from the previous time. She again responded well, her mental and physical symptoms all calming down rapidly after an initial aggravation.

Winter came and with it a new boyfriend. Peter was the brother of a good friend of Stella's, but they had somehow never crossed paths before. Stella told me that he was "sweet and thoughtful; he can't do enough for you, and there was an instant connection between us." She knew she was in love with him a month after they started dating. "After dating losers for so long," she said, "I have a well-developed 'Spidey sense,' and there is nothing about him that makes my sensitive Spidey senses tingle."

Spring came around, and Stella was sneezing up a storm, eyes and nose running—an attack of hay fever worse than she'd ever had. A quick course of low potency Allium alleviated these symptoms. Allium is made from onions which, of course, are famous for making your eyes sting and water.

Late in the summer, Stella was hit with large and unexpected bills:

her car died, and she needed expensive dental work. These events, along with the stress of her business struggling to become established, caused her fears about money to become acute, and she was worried about the long-term health of her teeth. The Arsenicum miasm was back yet again, with its characteristic anxiety over money and health. Stella took the next higher dose of Arsenicum, now only three levels from the highest possible potency. She survived the expected aggravation, during which she was even more anxious, ending up much calmer and more relaxed one week later.

A month later, I gave Stella Stellaria for rheumatic complaints that shifted from one joint to another. Stella's primary focus was on her business—she was determined to make it a success—but her wrists would bother her one day, the next it would be her knees. Bryonia is more typically called for in this type of situation, but Stella was not having headaches, which are characteristic of Bryonia, so I chose Stellaria. Within a few days of beginning the Stellaria, all of Stella's joints were better and she could focus on making her salon a success without distraction.

Three months later, Stella developed migraines. She was still very focused on her business; this time I gave her Bryonia, and the headaches resolved quickly. Stella also told me exciting news. Not only was her business stable and growing, but she was engaged! "This is the healthiest, best relationship I've ever been in," she said, glowing with happiness. "Peter is one of the kindest, most giving people I've ever met."

Reading this story and looking back over the years, Stella is impressed by her progress. "You can't see how stuck you are when you're in the middle of it. I seemed kind of pathetic there for a while, but I was! The changes are subtle at the time, and you don't realize how much you are changing, but looking back now, I can't believe how much I've changed!"

Chapter 4

Betty Lou

Betty Lou is an exuberant and loving, young at heart woman in her mid-fifties. There is no one better to tell your hopes and dreams, adventures and escapades to than Betty Lou. She will laugh with you till you're both doubled over and gasping for breath, sympathize to the point of tears in difficult times, and top it off with a warm hug and kiss. Betty Lou lives in the moment, and it serves her well in a life that has been full of challenges.

When I first met Betty Lou ten years ago, she was experiencing regular debilitating headaches, frequent nausea, hay fever, exhaustion, depression, and weight gain. We started with a very slow, careful buildup of time on a vibration machine. Partly because Betty had difficulty changing her diet, and also because I had only a powerful vibration machine at that time, we started with just fifteen seconds, at the lowest speed setting, several times a week. Even a tiny amount of vibration can have a large effect on a person's body and mind: at the end of six months we were still up to only a few minutes per session, but she was markedly better.

From the beginning, Betty Lou saw immediate and dramatic improvements in her energy level, mood, headaches, and digestive system, as long as we didn't do too much. Eventually, Betty began to see the connection between what she was eating and how she felt, and she started making wiser choices, which sped up her healing and allowed her to tolerate more vibration (see appendix 1).

In her own words, she had become "the Energizer Bunny." She could now mow the entire expanse of lawn behind her house, instead of just the small fraction of it she had been mowing earlier in the summer. Her hay fever, headaches, and nausea were all gone, and by the end of a year, she had lost thirty pounds. She was was amazing herself and her relatives with her energy. She told me about a family get-together at which they were all playing an informal game that involved a ball and a lot of running. She dominated the game, running up and down the field, blowing her relatives away.

After about two years of continued success, Betty Lou moved to Florida to help take care of her mother, who was elderly and ailing. I did not see her for the next six years. Eventually, Betty's mother passed on; then, a year later, her father died. Betty had devoted her life to her parents, so their deaths were hard for her, and her grief took its toll on her physical health.

By the time she returned to this area and contacted me, about two years ago, Betty's health was shaky again, and she had gained not only all the original weight back but also an additional ten to twenty pounds. Betty wanted to lose some weight, but it would not come off, no matter how little and well she ate or how much vibration and exercise she got. This time, Betty needed the help of homeopathic remedies along with her vibration and healthy eating program.

With homeopathy, you must treat whatever layer of negative energy is at the surface and expressing itself most acutely in the physical and emotional realms, following the body's wisdom and guidance as to what it needs. We could not start by off by directly addressing her desire to lose weight. Our body will prioritize what it needs; it will address the most critical health issues first, and it does not care what we look like. Luckily for us, though, the healthier we get, the better we do tend to look!

At this point in time, Betty's acute physical symptom was cystitis (an inflammation of the bladder and urinary tract, whether due to an infection or some other cause). I gave her Equisetum for low Kidney Fire due to the loss of her parents, a loss that was affecting Betty Lou's energy and health. With the Equisetum, Betty's cystitis cleared up in a few days.

Betty never did need a grief remedy, which may be because she is such an open and expressive person. Her emotions are strong and flow freely, to an extent that can be startling and unexpected for the more controlled people around her, but this openness helps her energy to stay clear.

Next I gave Betty Calcarea Carbonica, a classic remedy made from oyster shells and used for someone who is clinging to the security of home. The person who needs Calc Carb is typically "over-worked, over-burdened, and overwhelmed" by a "strong sense of duty and responsibility," and they can be obstinate.[1] Betty had been struggling hard to help all her loved ones, as well as herself, to stay afloat in a difficult world. It was not easy, and she had exhausted herself working at it. There had also been many arguments about uncooperative behavior from the loved ones she was trying to help, but she had not given up.

People in the Calc Carb state are also very often overweight. They have a tendency to "put on weight quickly and easily"[2] and have little desire for exercise and otherwise intense activities. "Calcarea is content to stay at home and watch television, preferably with someone to cuddle, and a good supply of high calorie nibbles."[3] Since negative characteristics associated with a remedy are likely to get better by letting go of that energy, Betty Lou's hormonal and metabolic imbalances that had caused her to gain weight and have difficulty losing it might now improve.

On the physical level, Betty had been having trouble with exhaustion, and she would end up out of breath after climbing a flight of stairs. Her lower back had also been hurting her enough that she had taken to wearing a back brace, all typical symptoms of Calc Carb. After a few days on the Calc Carb, Betty was not as tired or losing her breath as easily. Reversing her weight-gaining tendency would take longer, but we had begun the process with this remedy.

A month later, Betty's back pain came back, so I gave her low potency Rhus Toxicodendron for "cheerful, joking, and very lively" people who have joint problems, particularly arthritis and back pain.[4] With the Calc Carb energy released, her mood had improved, so she was now resonating to this new remedy. After a couple of days on the Rhus Tox remedy, Betty's pain was gone, though she was still wearing the back brace, just to be safe.

One week later, Betty's anxiety levels spiked. She was very worried about money. Her immediate problem was that she needed to move a great deal of her stuff, which had been in storage for many years, into a new storage unit. It was a big job, and she couldn't get anybody to help her—not surprisingly, there was a lack of enthusiasm for this project, as it had been a monthly event for years.

Betty had been hanging onto a large number of accumulated items from her past that had strong sentimental value but little current use-fulness. Friends and family had been trying to get her to dispose of her collection for years with no success. Every month she managed to move it, with the help of a truck and a sometimes bitterly complaining boyfriend, to another storage unit to take advantage of special, low-introductory rates.

I gave Betty Baryta Carbonica, a powerful remedy indicated for people who have a type of arrested emotional development often due to some type of childhood trauma. Baryta characteristics include: "Childish behavior. Needs reassurance. Easily influenced. Lack of self-confidence. . . . Extreme difficulty in making any decision. Anxiety disorder."[5] Betty's unbridled enthusiasm for life is a wonderful quality, but there is a childlike quality to her that holds her back. She sometimes asks for help when she is capable of handling a situation herself, such as the time she called me (vacationing on an island in Maine), very upset, to tell me she had been stung by a bee. "What should I do?" she asked me in a panic.

In a stunning turnaround, within a few weeks of starting a six-week course of high potency Baryta, Betty became a dynamo of enthusiasm for dumping and selling her childhood baggage. A valuable

Barbie doll collection went on eBay; reams of stuff made its way to a weekly flea market; and a fancy car, which she couldn't afford but had been hanging onto for many years because her father had given it to her, finally found another home. Overnight, Betty became a business dynamo, making savvy deals left and right.

One day she said to me, "I'm getting rid of a drum set my sister gave me twenty years ago. I don't even play the drums; I don't know why I've been hanging onto it for so long!" About the Cadillac Fleetwood from her father, she said, "I don't know why I didn't sell that car years ago. I can't afford to have three cars!" Betty barely had time to squeeze in her visits to me, such a fire of moving-forward energy had been lit under her. She would rush in and out of her appointments telling me, "I've got to go, there is so much to do. . . ."

About two months went by, full of flea markets and busy activity, till one day Betty told me that she had been wheezing again from another chest cold, a recurring problem for her—one that had even, on a few occasions, resulted in pneumonia. She also was exhausted again. Betty is a classic Phosphorus type person at heart, bright and bubbly, "like the bubbles from a carbonated drink," according to Bailey. He goes on to describe this personality as "the type that everyone wishes they belonged to."[6] But while certain Phosphorus characteristics can be highly appealing, this energy may still need tuning.

All homeopathic types have both positive and negative characteristics. The essence of Phosphorus is a lack of personal boundaries; like a bubble, Bailey describes this state of weak boundaries as leading to an incomplete ego and intellectual identification in childhood, such that "Phosphorus tends to experience the world like a young child. Sensory stimuli are more vibrant and immediate to Phosphorus, because they are not filtered by the intellect to the same degree as in others."[7]

Betty has always been extreme in her reactions to nearly everything. Small or large, new sounds, sights, and ideas elicit gasps of surprise and a thrill of excitement far beyond that of the average person. Phosphorus is probably Betty's true nature—her deepest energy, or "constitution."

I started her on a gentle but long-term program of Phosphorus that is particularly suited to the effects of a chronic situation.

Phosphorus is also famous for its effects on the lungs and well known for helping exhaustion: "Recurring respiratory infections; every cold goes to chest. Pneumonia. . . . Debility and collapse states."[8] Within a few days, Betty's wheezing had begun to clear up, and she was feeling stronger again, but she would stay on this program for at least six months to strengthen this constitutional energy so that she would no longer have a tendency for lung problems. On the psychological level, this program should also increase her ability to effectively create boundaries between herself and others.

Betty's next crisis came a month later when a brewing dispute with a neighbor in the rough section of the city where she and her boyfriend live came to a head. The tires on both of their cars were slashed late one night. Though they couldn't prove it, they were sure that this angry and vindictive neighbor had done it. They installed a security camera for possible future problems, but the police could do nothing about this incident, and Betty Lou and her boyfriend were left feeling angry and vulnerable.

I heard about this situation when Betty showed up limping; she had a severe pain in her ankle that had begun suddenly and had been going on for several days. She told me that nothing had happened to her foot, and she had no idea why she was in so much pain. I gave her Ruta Graveolens, famous for "injuries to tendons from strains or twisting of joints" in conjunction with "anxiety and panic disorders with fear of death."[9] The next day, Betty was no longer limping and her ankle pain was nearly gone. The underlying cause of Betty's ankle problem was the fear created by the slashed tires episode, so releasing this fear fixed her ankle.

One month later, Betty had a meltdown. Diffuse anxiety overwhelmed her, and she was in tears talking to me, despairing of her relationships, financial state, health—anything and everything. She was also itchy everywhere, a new symptom for her. I gave her one dose of Psorinum, a remedy used for eczema and tremendous itching accompanied by deep states of anxiety, hopelessness, and despair.[10] Within a week, Betty was back to her more optimistic and calmer self, and her itchiness was gone.

Since I first met Betty Lou, she has changed significantly. Her overall health is much stronger, and her ability to navigate a challenging world has increased. Anxiety, depression, and self-defeating behaviors are greatly decreased or gone. She has begun to lose weight again (ten pounds, so far), and her gifts of joy, enthusiasm, and empathy shine strongly, attracting others and strengthening herself. Growth is a process that never ends; homeopathy helps us to follow our true path with greater success.

Chapter 5

Marc

Marc is a professional man in his late forties who has always worked hard, persevering and succeeding despite challenges that began early in his life. When Marc was four years old, a car accident left him with a brain injury that caused complex partial seizures. Powerful drugs controlled this problem for many years, but they also resulted in drowsiness, fatigue, moodiness, and concentration and memory problems. Despite this, with much hard work and determination, Marc did well in school, eventually receiving a PhD in electrical engineering and working successfully in his field for the next twenty years.

When I met Marc in January 2013, he had been laid off, was searching for a new job, and was looking for a way to decrease his dose of Keppra, his antiseizure medication. For the previous eleven years, he had been on the highest possible dose (3,000 mg per day) and unable to lower that dose without the seizures returning. While the drugs did control his seizures, he had come to realize how much the drugs were also impacting his quality of life.

With his doctor's encouragement, he had been looking at alternative health methods to help control the seizures. Consulting *Alternative Therapies in Epilepsy Care,* by Devinsky, Schachter, and Pacia, he had identified homeopathic care as a natural therapy that might help him achieve his goal. Marc cannot do any whole body vibration, despite its known neurological stimulation and benefits, since seizures can be triggered by vibration.*

Marc had always been able to sense neurological disturbances, called "auras," within himself prior to a seizure, although he had been seizure free for eleven years. He described them with this analogy: the aura before a seizure is to a seizure as the feeling one has before a sneeze is to a sneeze. There was the feeling of something building within that sometimes comes to a climax but at other times recedes. When he tried to reduce his dose of Keppra, the auras would become more frequent and intense. He planned to use his ability to sense these auras as a way to safely reduce the drugs and judge the effectiveness of treatment.

The first homeopathic remedy I gave Marc was Cicuta, a classic remedy for seizures, particularly for "convulsions after head injuries . . . retardation after head injury."[1] He took one dose a week for twelve weeks. After each dose, he noticed an increase in the aura warning sensations before a calming effect signaled by a decrease in this monitoring sign. One might think the remedy was causing a worsening of his problem, except there was a general downward trend in the total number of the aura warning signs over time, and an initial "aggravation" is normal with high potency homeopathics.

A month after finishing this first three-month-long course of homeopathic treatment, Marc was able to successfully reduce his medication level to 2,250 mg per day, a 25 percent decrease from his starting point. The effects of a homeopathic remedy—that is, the action of that remedy on one's energy—are not fully complete until six to twelve months after taking the last dose, so there was hope that he would continue to improve over the next year.

Over the summer of 2013, Marc added neurofeedback, another therapy recommended by *Alternative Therapies in Epilepsy Care,* to his regimen. In the fall, following my recommendation, he began brain

---

*Some conditions are contraindicated for vibration. For a complete list of whole body vibration contraindications, go to http://www.BCVibrantHealth.com/whole-body-vibration/contraindications .php, or see my book, *Whole Body Vibration: The Future of Good Health.*

live-cell therapy, which provides nutrients and stimulation for repair and regrowth of damaged tissues (see appendix 2). When Marc was a child, magnetic resonance imaging had showed tissue damage to the brain, and this extra level of supplementation can be helpful in cases where an organ needs rejuvenation and regrowth. I also recommended a few other nutritional products to lower inflammation and support healing, such as omega-3 oils and a brain neurotransmitter–enhancement formula.

Since Marc had added several things at once to his program, it was hard to tell exactly what had caused what, but the characteristic pattern of aggravations after homeopathic remedies—where first one is markedly worse, then better—helped to confirm the action of the remedies. Using all of these therapies at the same time did give Marc the best chance of improvement, which was the primary goal, and all of these methods supported one another.

The homeopathy changed his energy, guiding his body and mind toward healing; nutrients are an essential component of healing, and ongoing retraining of his brain circuitry with neurofeedback also stimulates neurological change.

At this time, I also gave Marc two doses of Zincum in increasing potencies. Zincum is a remedy known for "tremendous excitation of the nervous system, which results in restlessness, abnormal or involuntary movements, twitches, and even convulsions."[2] Marc's medication level had recently dropped to 500 mg of Keppra per day, a dosage that was now more than 80 percent lower than his original level. With this drop, he developed twitches in his legs that were keeping him up at night. Zincum is a remedy for restless legs syndrome and "insomnia from restlessness or jerking,"[3] along with many other nervous system problems.

Marc noticed that his leg twitches would initially increase for a day or two after each dose of Zincum, during the aggravation period. They would then disappear, only to reappear, again less severely, shortly before he was due for his next dose. He also noticed a general improvement in his mental functioning after each dose. A year after we started, his overall quality of life had improved, especially the drowsiness and fatigue issues that had been caused by the high doses of Keppra.

In January 2014, Marc tried to lower his medications another level, to 250 mg per day, but he began to experience mini-seizures. These mini-seizures consisted of confusion and the inability to come up with certain words. They were not as intense as the seizures he'd had before he went on medication, but they were a sign that he could not yet reduce his medication to that level. He went back to 500 mg, and we continued with his program. In the spring of 2014, returning leg twitches signaled the surfacing of another layer of energy disturbance, and I gave him another dose of Zincum at the next higher potency level. Within days, he was resting comfortably.

By the end of that summer, Marc was down to 250 mg of Keppra per day, but he was complaining of difficulty focusing and concentrating, and he was having trouble sleeping. I gave him Graphites for "slow thinking, irresolution, poor concentration" in a "simple, basic, earthy" person.[4] Marc is a salt-of-the-earth kind of guy, hard-working and intelligent but not given to artistic flights of fancy. Graphites is also listed for "restlessness and anxiety at night,"[5] so it was likely his sleep would improve also. Within a few days, Marc reported to me that he was working well and sleeping comfortably.

A month or so later when I saw Marc, I could see that sadness that had been buried was coming to the surface. His struggle to survive had consumed his life, and his family had not been supportive. There was some problem from the past in his family that he had not talked about, but his pain had become more acute, along with the physical symptoms associated with this grief.

Marc needed Natrum Arsenicum, another variation of the classic Natrum "buried grief" remedy series; this one for someone who, along with grief, is "ambitious; super-achiever; practical; perfectionist."[6] I gave Marc a dose, and he reported to me that shortly afterward, for the first time in many years, he was suddenly more awake sexually and interested in women.

This is a classic reaction to Natrum remedies, which are known for "too serious and overly proper and responsible" people who, at heart, are "often highly romantic but after a disappointment, closes himself to further relationships for many years."[7] This situation can be due to any major loss, whether from divorce, death, or some other reason for a fractured family.

In December 2013, Marc was offered a new position with a company about an hour's drive away. With the stress of the new job, Marc found that he had to increase his meds one notch up from his most recent drop to 125 mg. Marc's doctor advised that he hold steady at the 250 mg level for the next several months while adjusting to his new job. Marc was now finished with the brain live-cell therapy and almost done with his neurofeedback program. We continued with the homeopathics in the hope that by the time he was ready to reduce his drugs further, it would be successful.

New jobs are challenging, and Marc was working hard to master the new information. Soon he needed Nux Vomica, for a person who is "irritable, impatient, ambitious and driven, workaholic."[8] Marc's sleep was problematic again, and Nux Vomica is associated with "insomnia, wakes especially at 3 or 4 am and cannot sleep due to thoughts about work."[9] A few days later, he was able to sleep, and though he was still working hard, he was effective without feeling stressed or irritated.

The next remedy was Tarentula Hispanica, for "over-activity and marked industriousness: workaholism."[10] Tarentula Hisp is sometimes used for hyperactivity in children and adults, and Marc's focus on work had become too intense. Marc had also developed a twitch in his eyelid. Tarentula Hisp is associated with twitching in general and specifically with eye twitches.[11] I gave him Tarentula Hisp at a low potency for a more surface-energy disturbance primarily expressing itself on the physical plane. When I saw him a month later, he reported that within a few days, his eye twitch was 90 percent better and that all month he worked well and had good focus and concentration.

The next remedy was Kali Carbonicum, for "conservative, loyal, moral, proper people," for whom it is "very difficult to express feeling, and he exercises strong control over his emotions."[12] This was a good description of Marc's personality, and on the physical level, Marc had been suffering from an upset stomach for the last two weeks. Kali Carb energy disturbances often include a fear of "diseases, especially that disease is about to appear (impending)," and they are often expressed in the gastric system.[13] I knew that Marc was worried that his neurological and medical issues might reappear and cause havoc with his new life and job.

Marc told me later that he noticed a pattern of a little worse, then better, after each of the three doses he took. Marc wisely takes his remedies on Fridays so that by Monday he will be back to his best state, ready for whatever comes his way.

Almost two years after he started with me, his medication level was down from the original 3,000 mg of Keppra a day to 250 mg, a drop of more than 90 percent, and Marc had a newfound energy and zest for life, plus a new job. He had finished with the brain live-cell therapy and the neurofeedback program several months earlier. Marc will continue with the homeopathics with the hope of soon not needing his Keppra medication at all.

Chapter 6

Christy

Christy is a dynamic and intuitive woman with a daredevil side. She's been training horses professionally and riding for many years, and you have to be tough, smart, and brave to handle a frightened, rampaging horse. She is sensitive in her work as well, which helps her to be effective. I once had a chance to observe her riding and working with her own horses, and I was impressed by her skill and connection to her animals. However, when I first met her, she was mired in frustration, anger, and worry.

Christy had recently gone out on her own, beginning her own business in her field after working for others for many years. She had been working for an organization run by a man she respected, but the situation had become intolerable, and she had quit about six months before I met her. She was still angry and bitter, and I heard all about it—the gist being that the workplace dynamics had led to favoritism, acrimony, and backstabbing, which had created an intolerable work environment.

Christy's primary focus at that time was on money and her fledgling business. She was feeling uptight about the sudden lack of income and the need to find a new source of clients in a small field. She also mentioned that there had been no men in her life for quite a few years and that she would like to change the situation, but "there just aren't any decent men out there!"

Christy believes in the power of energy, and she primarily came to me for help moving her life forward. She is quite a healthy person over-all, having just a few minor physical issues. Her energy level was lower than it had once been, there were a couple of digestive discomforts, the beginnings of a bone-density issue, and occasional back pain.

Christy had tried whole body vibration with me a few times and loved the effects she'd noticed, but money was tight, so she was holding off on any big purchases. She decided to just stick to the homeopathics for the moment.

The first homeopathic I gave Christy was a dose of Lachesis, for "passionate, intense people. . . . Jealousy. Envy. Suspicion, even para-noia. Loquacity. Anger. Aggressiveness."[1] Christy had been immersed in her difficult work situation for some time, and it was bringing these qualities in her psyche to the surface. I had also barely gotten a word in myself during our first hour-long meeting, so the hallmark signs of Lachesis (loquacity and anger) were clear.

Lachesis is also one of the most sexually passionate types; "like a highly strung bow, . . . the Lachesis individual vibrates with sexual energy."[2] But this energy "must find an outlet if it is not to backfire on its owner."[3] While Christy is a passionate person, she has been frus-trated in her love life.

Thirty minutes after Christy's first dose of Lachesis, she told me that a strange taste and foamy sensation in her mouth, which had been bothering her for weeks, was suddenly gone. Christy never did expe-rience an "aggravation" with this remedy, she only got better. She is one of the lucky few who just gets better from a high potency remedy, at least most of the time. After a few days, Christy had burgeoning energy for building her business and for life in general. Her digestive issues and her back were also better.

By the end of a week, Christy was reporting a sense of calm and well-being. In a conversation during which I could finally get a word in edgewise, I heard nothing about the old work situation, only positive things about her health improvements and new ideas she'd had for promoting her business.

Several months after her first consult, Christy returned with the same signs and symptoms as before, though slightly less intense. It often takes several doses of the same remedy at gradually increasing potencies to fully let go of an entrenched energy. I gave her another dose of Lachesis, one potency level up. Christy had a very similar reaction: immediate physical changes, followed by calming and focusing effects and a letting go of anger and resentment.

A few months later, as summer was approaching, Christy came back full of anxiety and fear. Her finances were shaky, and she was afraid she might lose her house. She had no security, and it seemed nearly impossible to find more clients. Her family was of little help, busy as they were with their own lives, not recognizing her talents, and not particularly supportive of her in general. Christy felt hopeless and despairing, like no matter what she did, the situation would not change.

Christy has a family history of osteoporosis and has developed osteopenia herself; her back pain had come back, and she was experiencing headaches, which were unusual for her. I gave Christy a remedy called Syphilinum, which is associated with great fear and anxiety along with a "type of nihilism or a feeling to let everything crash down around him" and "a tendency for a lack of strong connection with others."[4] Syphilinum is also characteristically associated, on the physical level, with "erosions of the bone . . . back pain . . . headache."[5]

Syphilinum is one of the most powerful negative energies, the releasing of which is likely to trigger great change—and it did. When I next heard from Christy, she called to tell me what a fantastic summer she'd had. Her work had picked up, suddenly getting several new clients. Plus two guys had appeared in her life, and she had been busy dating both, trying to decide which one was best for her.

One of the guys was a wild and intense person, which was exciting, but he was also immature and self-centered. The other man was a new experience for Christy. Sensitive and kind, mature, intelligent, and secure, he treated her with thoughtful care and consideration.

They were enjoying boating adventures up and down the New England coast, rapidly becoming the best of friends as well as lovers. It wasn't long before she decided that this was not a difficult choice. She didn't need another crazy relationship. Derek was touching her heart, and there was long-term potential there.

However, Christy also told me that while Derek was loving and warm much of the time, telling her how wonderful she was and how much he cared for her, he also subtlety pushed her away at times. Eight months prior, Derek had lost his wife of ten years after caring for her throughout a long illness. Christy's friends warned her to watch out for the rebound effect and the Internet had confirmed this; men who start dating soon after the death of a spouse are bad bets, either emotionally unavailable or having other issues that surface later on.

Christy convinced her new boyfriend to come with her for a consultation with me. Derek was open-minded and impressed me with his strength and thoughtfulness. He had never heard of homeopathy before Christy began telling him about her experiences, but he was willing to see what it was all about. They had also been talking about whole body vibration, and they had decided to buy a machine together.

At this point, Christy was able to start vibrating more frequently and regularly, and there was sudden increase in how many homeopathics she needed. This follows the pattern I have discussed before: vibration seems to increase the rate of energy change. Initially, she had needed a new remedy every two to three months; after beginning to vibrate, that rate jumped to almost once a month.

Christy had not been feeling well again, and she wanted another dose of that Syphilinum remedy. "I've never felt so good," she said, "give me more!" But a remedy has to be exactly the right remedy, resonating to the energy currently at the surface, and this time the situation was different. Christy had developed an irritating rash, she was tired, and she was preoccupied with making sure she was covering every angle in her business, dotting all the i's and crossing every t.

I gave her a dose of Kali Sulfuricum, which combines the characteristic Kali need to "follow rules to the smallest detail,"[6] and Sulfur's outgoing, extroverted, friendly, passionate personality who has a tendency for skin issues.

After talking with Derek, I felt that he was still grieving for his wife, though he was not aware of it; he had blocked the grief because it was so painful. He did not allow himself to fall apart, as he had many responsibilities and people depending on him. I gave him a dose of Natrum Carbonicum, for a "gentle, refined, selfless" person who has blocked "sadness and grief" with a "cheerful demeanor."[7] Physically, Derek was a healthy, active guy, but his shoulders slumped under the heavy weight of responsibility he always carried, and Nat Carb is associated with "stoop-shoulders."[8]

A few days later, I heard from Christy. Unusually for her, with Kali Sulf she'd had an aggravation. Starting the morning after taking the remedy and lasting for several days, she was suddenly weak and exhausted, tired just from climbing the stairs to her house, which was a strange experience for her.

A month or so later I heard from Christy again. She was falling in love! She told me how warm and tender Derek was, how he treated her better than anybody had ever treated her, how he would tell her how much he cared for her, and how special she was to him. She said that Derek loved her wild side. All of his life, Derek had been the responsible one, taking care of the people around him; Christy was exciting and exotic for him, a breath of fresh air.

I heard about more boating adventures and the Topsfield Fair, where they and another friend had all tried a big powerful vibration machine that was being shown and sold at the expo. Everybody had a grand time trying the machine, laughing hysterically at the new sensations, but Christy's friend ended up ill the next day. Too much vibration, especially without building up gradually, can cause problems.*

A month later, I heard from Christy once more. This time she told

---

*Whole body vibration has many powerful beneficial effects on the body, mind, and spirit, but the powerful detoxification effect, while good in moderation, can also stress your body and aggravate symptoms if you do too much too soon. Also, there are quite a few contraindications (health situations that are likely to get worse with vibration), so people should check these out before trying vibration. For a complete list, check my website, www.BCVibrantHealth.com, or my book, *Whole Body Vibration: The Future of Good Health.*

me, *at length*, how Derek had been better for a while, but now he was back to his old tricks; one day he was warm and loving, the next he was pushing her away. It was subtle, but she is sensitive and got the message. Christy was angry and not sure he was the right guy for her. She wanted a guy who was ready for a committed relationship, she said, not this "maybe yes, maybe no" scenario. I gave Christy one more dose, one potency level higher, of Lachesis for anger, sexual tension, and loquaciousness.

As the holidays approached, Christy was stressed out and irritable. She was trying to help her father, who'd had a reoccurrence of cancer, and take care of her business, which was getting busier. The prognosis for her father was not hopeful, though they were trying radiation treatments.

Christy had had a childhood full of criticism from her father. She felt that whatever she did, it was never good enough. Though he has apologized for the past and is grateful for her help these days, she is still sensitive to his now rare criticism.

I gave Christy Sepia, a classic remedy for "the independent woman"[9] who is "careworn . . . irritable . . . disconnected . . . from family."[10] Also matching are Christy's relationships and interactions with men; Sepia "tends to be herself, rather than try to conform or please. . . . is often a puzzle to men, who are either fascinated by her mystery, or leave her well alone."[11]

The next time I heard from Christy, two weeks later, disaster had struck—with a boom. A perfect storm had hit Derek: the confluence of the anniversary of his wife's death, the stress of the holiday season, and his usual troubles with Seasonal Affective Disorder. In a spasm of grief, he had showed up at Christy's house one evening to tell her that he "didn't know if he could ever love another woman as much as he had loved his first wife," and he needed more space.

Christy was devastated, though she had held it together while he was there. She'd had a sleepless night full of tears and rage, and the next day she'd gone through a storage room, "cleaning it in a whirlwind, stomping on boxes and throwing things in all directions." Christy had begun to trust and believe in a man again. She had been in love for the first time in many years, only to have this love ripped away.

I gave Christy Natrum Phosphoricum for grief in a person who combines the classic buried grief and depression of all Natrum remedies with the sympathy and fears of Phosphorus. While she was angry at Derek, I felt that this current grief, unearthed by the pain of Derek's rejection, was related to her original buried grief over her father's inability to express his love for her.

Derek is an intelligent and caring guy who did not want to hurt Christy, but he was overwhelmed by his own grief. He recognized that he had been waffling with Christy, felt bad about it, and agreed to come see me again. Derek was dealing with the same situation as before, so I gave him another, higher potency dose of Nat Carb, his particular flavor of the many possible flavors of Natrum, along with a warning that he was likely to feel worse before he felt better.

Derek and Christy had been planning, before their relationship crisis, to go on a week-long vacation together in the Caribbean at the end of January. Now the trip was up in the air, though the tickets were already bought. Christy understood Derek's grief and his need for space, but she vowed never to let him get close again, never to let him have such power over her. I advised Christy to give the situation some time to calm down, knowing that once they had gotten through the aggravation periods of their remedies, the situation was likely to improve.

A week or so later, Christy called me; she was no longer sad, now she was angry! She talked fast, letting off steam about the situation with Derek. "How can you compete with memories?!"

However, she and Derek had been communicating; Derek had apologized for his hurtful outburst, and he was sympathetic to her feelings. Neither one of them was ready to give up on their relationship; in fact, they both still wanted to go on vacation together. I gave Christy one more dose, now at a very high potency, of Lachesis. At this level, the effect would reach deep into her psyche and would be very powerful.

Two days later Christy called—she was in the middle of an aggravation. "I'm angry at the world, and I just can't stop talking a mile a minute!" She had been getting lots of new clients lately, she said, "but I'm afraid to call them back! I'm going to take an anti-anxiety pill and call them later." I was encouraged, feeling that this might be the final release of this nasty energy disturbance.

Two weeks later I heard from an ebullient Christy. She and Derek had had a "phenomenal, off the charts vacation! My honeymoon wasn't this good!" One day they had gotten stuck driving through isolated dunes in a rented jeep and made it out by working together. Derek had stayed calm, focused, and steadfast and had listened to her suggestions, which had impressed Christy and increased her trust in him.

They went dancing under the moon and drank shots of whiskey, exuberant and uninhibited. Derek had told her, "This is the best vacation I've ever had!" He also told her that when he went to his next grief counseling group meeting, he was going to tell them, "Stop wallowing in your past. I've found a wonderful woman, and I'm moving on!"

One week after that, Christy's father was dying of cancer. She told me, nonstop for twenty minutes, about the trouble and difficulties she was having in her life. There was a cold, unsympathetic, angry edge to her voice as she told me how she tried to help people, but it seemed impossible sometimes. Even her newly back-in-grace boyfriend did not escape unscathed—as he was now back in his noncommittal, blowing hot and cold state.

I gave her another dose of Sepia, for "the independent woman" who has become "hard and indifferent . . . disconnected,"[12] in response to mistreatment and pain. This Sepia remedy would help Christy let go of the pain inside her that was the source of the walls her psyche had constructed long ago.

Regarding Derek, she told me that he needed time, that he was in a process of exploring his independence after a lifetime of responsibilities, but she didn't know if she wanted to wait around for him. She wanted a man who was ready to commit. She'd tried to get him to come see me again, but he was reluctant.

"I don't know what Becky did," he'd told her, "but something came over me with that last remedy. I couldn't control it, and I went into this big funk!" Derek had had an aggravation reaction, which can cause an increase in emotional and physical symptoms. Not understanding this process, however, it had scared him.

I reminded Christy that it can take at least six months for a homeopathic remedy to fully act and for the energy to change. "Don't worry," I said, "your energy will be so positive that lots of men, including Derek, will be attracted to you—and you can choose whichever one you want."

When I called Christy a month later to talk about including her story in this book, she told me how wonderful things were for her these days. She was very busy with her work. There were lots of new clients and money coming in, which was gratifying and provided security, and her relationship with Derek was "fantastic."

She had been in an accident a few weeks earlier. The sight of her lying injured on the ground caused Derek to suddenly realize how important she was to him, and their relationship had taken a sudden turn for the better. Christy sees big changes in both of them, and feels the homeopathic remedies are part of what helped them both to change so dramatically. Christy was talking a mile a minute, but there was no anger; she was just high on happiness, and it was beautiful to see.

Chapter 7

My Story:
A Radical Approach

For twenty years, I worked with Dr. Keith DeOrio, a medical doctor who uses many natural health methods, including homeopathy. He treated me using a modern approach to homeopathy in which multiple remedies are used over time, often building up a particular remedy through several potency levels. Originally, I took three to five high potency homeopathic remedies per year. This number increased to ten to fifteen per year after I started using the proper type of whole body vibration (see chapter 2). This is also the method I used with the four clients whose stories I told in chapters 3 through 6.

Several years ago, I no longer needed to consult with Dr. DeOrio, as I had become experienced, knowledgeable, and intuitive enough to guide my own care and choose the correct homeopathic remedies myself. However, two years ago, my symptoms began to intensify; some earlier ones returned or increased in severity, and new ones appeared. Since then, I have used more than 230 high potency remedies, alternating doses of up to ten different homeopathics at a time, as I worked my way up from low potency doses to extremely high levels. Each time, I would experience an aggravation, which is the sudden worsening of symptoms, followed by rapid improvement. This effect gave me confidence that I was on the right track.

The type of homeopathic treatment I describe in this chapter is unheard of. You are not supposed to use more than one high potency homeopathic at a time, and not so many high potency remedies in total.* I believe that in my case, deep psychological issues resulting from a traumatic childhood combined with a sensitive nature, which led to many energy disturbances. This eventually led to a major health challenge.

Because I have been using whole body vibration and homeopathy for many years, my electromagnetic energy is very strong and vibrates at a high frequency. This allowed for very rapid energy change. Almost as fast as I would release one layer of negative energy with a homeopathic remedy, another layer would rise to the surface—much more rapidly than would usually happen—because of the electromagnetic effects of the whole body vibration (as described in chapter 2).

Admittedly, this is only theory at this point, but my many, often severe, symptoms are gone, and it was a clear step-by-step process. After a harrowing two years marked by a barrage of often debilitating symptoms, which would reliably worsen and then improve with the indicated homeopathic, I now have no symptoms at all. I am now feeling better than I have ever felt on every level: physical, mental, spiritual, and in my personal and professional life. It is hard to argue with success; that is why I'd like to see research in this area.

I don't expect other people to try this type of approach, as it is neither researched nor taught in schools of homeopathy. But I didn't just arbitrarily decide to take so many remedies at such high potencies. In an effort to heal myself, I followed my body's wisdom as shown by my symptoms. We each have our own destiny. Mine seems to be to explore the outer edges of natural health and report back my findings.

There is a long history of scientific innovations coming from people experimenting on themselves, including the founder of homeopathy

---

*It is common these days to take multiple low potency remedies at the same time, but not the high potency versions. There are, in fact, many combination low potency mixtures available in retail stores. Low potency remedies are usually taken several times per day, whereas high potency remedies are given much less often, sometime as only one dose once in a lifetime.

himself, Dr. Samuel Hahnemann. Benjamin Franklin nearly electrocuted himself while discovering electricity by experimenting with lightning, and Jonas Salk inoculated himself and all his family to test the polio vaccine he had created. I can't say that I experimented on myself for science and the betterment of mankind, as these people were doing. I did it because I felt this was my best chance for healing my myriad symptoms. The results speak for themselves.

I was quite ill, and I consulted with an allopathic medical doctor, but as is typical for me, Western medicine could not find anything to explain my symptoms. My doctor wanted to give me birth control pills to suppress my most alarming symptom, severe prolonged menstrual bleeding; but in the past, birth control pills have led to further problems for me. Birth control pills also would not have done anything for all the other symptoms I was experiencing. Remembering my successes with homeopathy in the past, I felt my best option was to follow my body's wisdom by treating my symptoms with homeopathic remedies.

While I realize that one person's experience, however remarkable, is not sufficient as convincing scientific evidence, I hope that my experience and this book will inspire further research and interest in homeopathy. The following is an account of this intense eighteen-month period in my life.

Becky's Story: Mothers and Daughters

A crescendo of energy change, like a fireworks finale, happened for me from 2014 to well into 2015. The previous year, I had been taking two to three homeopathics each month (thirty-one in total that year), many of them high potency, to heal a number of stubborn health issues. By February 2014, I was taking eight different homeopathics, most of them through eight levels of increasing strengths, starting low and ending at their highest potencies. With each remedy, I would have an aggravation, which indicated I was on the right track.

My main symptoms included a protracted cold and a sinus infection, as well as fluctuating joint and nerve pains, irritability, fatigue, itchy skin, allergies, eye pain and irritation, and the prolonged heavy menstrual bleeding mentioned earlier. These symptoms would come and go, along with others, as I continued to take different homeo-pathics of graduating intensity. The process was exhausting but also exciting and inspiring, as I felt it had the power to bring me to a fulfilling and healthy future. Rather than treating myself with pills that suppress symptoms, I was using the symptoms as signposts in my quest to heal my energy, which was the source of my disease.

One homeopathic I had been taking was Arsenicum Album. This remedy is famous for "tremendous anxiety . . . panic attacks . . . fear of disease . . . poverty."[1] Phillip Bailey, MD, sums up this energy with the keynote symptom of "physical insecurity."[2] It is also linked to fourteen-day cycles and a "hemorrhagic tendency" along with myr-iad physical symptoms. Most recently, I took the highest possible dose of this remedy, which, over the course of the next year, should fully release the last vestiges of this negative energy from my system.

According to the Law of Attraction,* by releasing insecurity about my physical safety and security (and thus this remedy's well-known fear of poverty), Arsenicum Album would help with my money prob-lems as well as my physical health. I did not expect immediate change in this area though, as it takes six to twelve months to fully see the effects of a high potency homeopathic remedy.

I was also taking Thuja, for "feelings of worthlessness . . . unat-tractiveness . . . depression . . . desperation to 'fit in,' and loneliness and sadness from a sense of being separate."[3] On the physical level, Thuja is associated with allergies, arthritis, rheumatism, and neuralgia, all of which I had. This mental state was rooted in my childhood depression.

The night after I started this remedy, during the aggravation, my knees were throbbing with pain. I was not discouraged; it was a posi-tive sign that the remedy was correct, and I would soon feel better.

---

*The Law of Attraction describes the phenomenon of attracting the same energy that one ema-nates. Acclaimed author Louise Hay is considered the mother of positive thinking. She states: "The Law of Attraction is that our thinking creates and brings to us whatever we think about." http://www.oprah.com/spirit/The-Law-of-Attraction-Real-Life-Stories_1#ixzz2ZKkusGCY (as of July 18, 2013).

In early May, I was still deep in the storm of homeopathics: nine high potency remedies each month for three months. Most recently, I'd had another three weeks of heavy menstruation that required the next highest potency of all four of the hemorrhaging remedies I was using.

Homeopathy and vibration, plus the stimulus and challenges of daily living, led to accelerated change. I think it was the vibration therapy that was accelerating the process so dramatically. Energetically attuned people talk about a global acceleration of energy that affects our whole world, but I took homeopathics for more than twenty years before I started vibration therapy, with little change in the process. Since vibrating, I have needed homeopathics at an ever-increasing rate; but along with my physical symptoms changing, I've also seen my abilities, achievements, and quality of life improving—beyond anything I could have imagined.

Through the summer of 2014, I continued on this course. At the end of October, I was becoming more concerned about the menstrual bleeding. I had begun a new remedy, Picricum. Its effects are centered on the spine (my back had been bothering me), and the "generative organs,"[4] which would include the womb. It is also linked to exhaustion and weakness, all typically (in this energy disturbance) caused by mental exertion and a fear of failure.[5] After the first dose, I was much worse. Suddenly, I was bleeding so heavily that I could not stop the flow even with two super-plus tampons inserted at the same time.

I had not gone to a medical doctor, as I'd had a complete medical workup two years earlier because of the heavy bleeding and severe associated pain that would not abate even with maximum doses of OxyContin. The doctors could not find anything wrong, ending up with an official diagnosis of "unexplainable pelvic area pain." I continued at the time with my homeopathic treatments and eventually eliminated the pain, but the bleeding continued to worsen.

The doctors had offered me birth control pills two years earlier to control the bleeding and pain, but I had used them as a young woman, and side effects were part of what led to me developing so many problems in the first place. Plus, birth control pills would not heal my many other symptoms. Instead, I was using the bleeding to help me know which homeopathic remedy I needed. In this way, I'd hoped to fix all of my ailments.

The bouts of heavy bleeding were triggered by movement and aggravations from the homeopathics, with all the major bleeding episodes coming shortly after one or the other. Exercise should not cause this kind of bleeding. The exercise was a trigger for some physical issue caused by the deeper energy issues. The homeopathics were releasing stuck negative energy, which leads to true healing, but this is also a stressful event for the body and mind, hence the aggravations.

Ten days after the first dose of Picricum, I took another, stronger dose. Five hours later, at a cocktail party, after nothing more vigorous than standing around talking to people, I began to bleed heavily again. Ten minutes into a conversation with a group of people, I blurted, "I've got to go!" and dashed off, successfully averting an awkward scene. It was clear this bleeding had to stop. I began to consider a consult with an allopathic doctor.

I went to a gynecologist, who was concerned, and she planned a full diagnostic workup. The first blood tests results all came back normal; I was not even anemic. This impressed the doctor, despite my iron rich diet, since the heavy bleeding, sometimes for more than a month at a time, had been going on for more than a year, and I had only occasionally taken half (due to uncomfortable side effects) a low-dose iron supplement pill. I did, however, take homeopathic Ferrum, which is a classic remedy for anemia. I was curious to see the results of the ultrasound my doctor had scheduled.

Meanwhile, I had an enlightening, though painful, experience with a friend I had known for many years. She is warm and kind most of the time, but if I talk to her when I am angry and upset, she is likely to take my generalized frustration and impatience at these times personally, due to her own history of trauma, and respond with a sharp attack. When I spoke to her, I was due for another dose of Causticum, famous for a mental state of "great anger over injustices."[6] Consequently, I was full of anger, though it had nothing to do with her directly. She picked up on the angry vibes immediately, though, and it triggered her. I felt betrayed, not cared about.

Victor, a dear friend of mine, pointed out that I was viewing my friend as my mother and that this was why this scenario had upset me so much. It is true—we carry our past with us, especially our childhoods and first attachments, and it colors our present. This incident was a hint that there was still trouble buried deep in my mind from my childhood problems with my mother.

Just before Christmas 2014, my mother was diagnosed with cancer. When she told me this, I did not react to her news in a normal way. I expressed sympathy and concern but felt little real emotion; then forgot about the whole thing. Hours later, I realized that I had not thought about her again all day. I realized then that I must not have fully forgiven her for the past.

Her diagnosis was not a complete surprise. Her doctors had been watching her for years, suspecting multiple myeloma, a blood and bone marrow cancer. She also was not in great distress herself, feeling that she'd had a long and good life (she was almost ninety years old), and that "nobody lives forever, so what difference does it make which way you go." However, I had simply forgotten about it minutes after being told, which was strange—and cold.

I realized then that I needed Aurum Muriaticum Naturatum—a remedy that combines the characteristics of Aurum and Natrum remedies. Together, they form a remedy that has powerful effects on the womb. Aurum is famous for "its ability to cure the deepest imaginable depressions and suicidal states . . . people who are very intense, idealistic, and who want to be the best and set high goals."[7] All Natrum remedies (there are several versions) are known for "ailments from grief and disappointed love. Silent grief. Dwells on past griefs . . . highly sensitive . . . wounds are deeply felt and result in the patient placing a psychological wall around himself to avoid further pain."[8]

The combination remedy of Aur Mur Nat is used when there are elements of both of these mental states, but, according to Morrison (homeopathic physician and author of several well-known homeopathic texts), the main pathology is uterine troubles. Some homeopaths also consider it to be the most important remedy for malignancies of the uterus.[9] My ultrasound results had come back with nothing to account for the abnormally heavy menstrual bleeding lasting for three months straight. The doctor had now scheduled me for a biopsy in January.

I felt it was not a coincidence that both my mother and I might be dealing with cancer at the same time, because we have been linked, from when I was in the womb, by a bond of pain and love. My illness was rooted in the sadness of a little girl who felt that her mother did not love her. For me to heal myself, I would need to fully forgive my mother. Pain and fear is a cancer in the soul that I believe can lead to cancer in the body.

Natrum remedies are known in homeopathy for their ability to heal deep and ancient griefs, especially grief and loss with respect to the mother. Mothers are supposed to provide the child with unconditional love; when they do not, the child suffers from a lack of emotional nourishment, and the remedy is Natrum.

I had blocked my mother out of fear, a fear so great that I had not even been aware of it. My fear was of annihilation, but it was based in what happened in the past, not the present. There was never any physical abuse, but emotionally my birth brought to the surface pain from her childhood. The result was a conflict in her between loving me and anger and pain redirected at me. Children are sensitive to energy and emotions, and I incorporated her negative messages into my psyche and body, which led to a lifetime of physical and emotional problems.

But I was mostly healed and strong by this time, and my mother had also matured and mellowed. She had been trying for many years to show me love, and to find love and forgiveness in return. I could see this on an intellectual level, but in blocking pain, I had blocked everything. She showed her love by supporting me in a great many ways, yet I could not feel it.

Several days after taking the Aur Mur Nat remedy, I was more peaceful. I felt I would be able to forgive my mother. When I meditated on the situation, I saw an image of a rabbit, an elderly mother rabbit.

It was my mother, the core of who she was at the time. Rabbits, with their fecundity, are symbolic of motherhood and babies, and my mother's children and grandchildren were her main focus then.

I focused on the rabbit's teeth, seeing them as large and prominent, but they were for eating not harming; a rabbit is about as harmless an animal as can be found. I also saw big, long ears waggling about. My mother was still on the alert for danger, more so than she needed to be. This was because of her unresolved guilt and hidden past, but big ears are also symbolic of wisdom, as listening is a key element of wisdom.

My mother and I spent New Year's Eve together, going out for dinner and a movie. I was taking baby steps toward trying to reach a more open state of communication with her. We had never been able to talk about or acknowledge the truth of what had happened when I was a very little child, and no one in my family knows of either my early experience with my mother or her hidden past.

My mother had reasons, based in her own childhood trauma, for how she had mistreated me when I was young. She was kind to me now, though, helping in me in many ways, and for me to get well, I needed to forgive her for the past.

She had been the one to come up with a plan for me to take care of my father during the last years of his life, paying me generously for this help, and giving me ongoing financial support. She has also helped me with my writing—editing manuscripts and paying for the cost of publishing my first books. She is always available to talk and makes an effort to be supportive of my ideas, however strange they may seem to her. She cooks up a storm, knits piles of sweaters, and takes care of the new babies in our family, generally doing her best to be a loving parent and grandmother. It was I who needed to change.

In mid-January, I heard from my doctor that the biopsy was negative—I did not have cancer. They had found some sort of growth, but it was benign. Western medicine had ended up with no explanation for either my original symptoms or their current disappearance.

I wondered if I'd had cancer but that I'd healed myself with homeopathics and vibration therapy before the biopsy was done. The bleeding had actually been tapering off during the month before the biopsy, and I had by now stopped bleeding entirely. Many of the remedies that I took are famous for their anticancer effects, and Aur Mur Nat is famous for uterine malignancies, considered by some homeopaths to be the most powerful remedy for this type of cancer.*

I had been very sick during 2014, much sicker than I should have been, with exhaustion and signs of immune system distress, as well as the bleeding. I'd also suffered intense pain from menstruation for many years. A natural health medical doctor, who specializes in energy medicine, once told me that extreme pain of that nature, over a long period of time, would likely lead to cancer. Whether I'd averted cancer or not, I *was* healing all the miserable symptoms I had been struggling with for years, and that is what was most important.

I think that my many years of vibration and homeopathy strengthened my body and energy to the point that I could endure taking what eventually came to a final total of 230 high potency remedies over an eighteen-month period.† Some classical homeopaths still believe you should give a person only one high potency remedy ever in their entire lifetime, though many homeopaths now do use multiple remedies over time.

In February 2015, one year after my crescendo of energy change began, my body was better. There had been no bleeding for more than a month, and I was outdoors shoveling snow for hours some days (there were numerous back-to-back major snowstorms in New England in 2015) and feeling great. My mother was also doing well, though she was easily fatigued. The chemo side effects were not expected to be bad with her particular drugs, and her doctors were

---

*More than half the remedies I took were either known to heal uterine cancer or were remedies for cancer in general. I was using them for other issues, but they would have also been treating cancer if I'd had it. Research conducted at MD Anderson, the top-ranked cancer hospital in the United States, has demonstrated the effectiveness of homeopathic remedies against cancer cells (see PubMed 20043074). For a survey of scientific research regarding homeopathy and cancer, including a discussion of clinical studies and state-of-the-art laboratory studies, see the 2009 article, "The Evidence: Scientific Studies on Homeopathic Cancer Treatment," by Manfred Mueller, MA, RSHom(NA), CCH. Available on the North American Society of Homeopaths website: https://www.homeopathy.org/portfolio-view/the-evidence-scientific-studies-on-homeopathic-cancer-treatment/ (as of July, 2015).
†The two hundred–plus number is counting different potencies of the same remedy, but not multiple doses of the same remedy at the same potency.

optimistic of an outcome that would give her five to seven more good-quality years.

I also felt full of love for myself, a wonderful state to be in. I felt toward myself as I felt for Sugar, my darling dog. When I caught sight of myself in a mirror, I would think to myself, "I love you!" It's not that I didn't see things I wanted to change, but I knew that I would change them over time in my desire to protect and take good care of myself.

By the spring of 2015, I was exercising two hours every other day, biking to a nature sanctuary in nearby Concord. I felt good, no joint problems, good energy, enjoying the sun and beauty of the world around me. I had lost about five pounds, plus I was toning up, so my clothes fit better. I love that feeling when you can just bounce up the stairs: slim, sleek, and svelte.

In June, my mother ended up in the ER again because of a sudden flare-up of back pain, a common symptom of her cancer. I was anxious and upset and thought about her all day, as opposed to my disconnected reaction when she had first told me her cancer diagnosis. My worried state was a sign of the progress we had made. Shortly after my mother recovered from the back-pain episode, which turned out to be unrelated to the cancer and easily resolved, I showed her this story. She reacted with love and acceptance, and we continue to build on the good from the past, letting go of pain and trouble.

One of the remarkable results of high potency homeopathy, which acts on the mental state as well as the physical, is that your mental state changes without any particular effort on your part beyond taking the homeopathic. As the energy releases, your thoughts and emotions will also shift. The biggest release typically happens within a few days of taking the remedy. I did experience this sudden shift, as seen with my suddenly increased peacefulness regarding my mother, a few days after taking the remedy. This process of releasing energy then continues at a slower rate for another six to twelve months. By four months after I took the Aur Mur Nat, there had been a major shift in my emotions and reactions regarding my mother.

Another example of the long-term effects of homeopathic remedies can be seen with the remedy Arsenicum Album, which I took at the beginning of my story. Its keynote mental state, "physical insecurity,"[10] is a first chakra issue of survival, of feeling safe and secure in a family where your physical needs will be met. This is something I did not have as a small child. I felt excluded, unwanted, and for most of my life it seemed that this sense of insecurity, especially in groups of people, would remain with me forever, but with the help of homeopathy and whole body vibration, that has all changed.

First chakra issues are also correlated with problems of the feet and legs, reflecting a lack of grounding, since your feet and legs are your physical connection to the ground. The first chakra is known as the root chakra; your family is your root, that which grounds you. I have had endless problems with my feet, ankles, knees, and hips, now all much better. It was one year after that final dose of Arsenicum that I had also achieved a greater level of economic security and a higher level of comfort and security within my family.

As this book goes into production, the bleeding is over. For a while it returned, though lighter, and there had been reoccurrences of other symptoms in lessening severity, but I continued to take homeopathic remedies to heal them. I am happy to say that I seem to be done at this point. I feel fantastic, have no symptoms at all, and am not currently taking any homeopathics. I am enjoying life as never before. I will keep a close eye on my body, and if it tells me that I need to fine-tune my energy again, I will do so. Tuning my energy is a process that not only helps my physical and mental health, but also helps me follow my true path in life.

Epilogue

My purpose in writing this book has been to bring the power of energy medicine to people worldwide who need and want help to change their lives. Homeopathy addresses body, mind, and spirit; thus it leads to a more complete cure than Western medicine alone can provide. As Plato said several centuries before Christ, but with a truth that still echoes today:

> The cure of the part should not be attempted without treatment of the whole. . . . If the head and body are to be healthy you must begin by curing the mind . . . the greatest error of our day in the treatment of the human body [is] that physicians separate the soul from the body.[1]

Dare to dream and be inspired. The world is waiting for you to fan to a bright flame the brilliant spark of energy that you already are. I hope that I have given you both a method and inspiration.

Gut Flora Imbalances

Our bodies are designed to have billions of beneficial microbes in our guts that help us to digest our food properly. Our modern lifestyles, however, do not support a healthy balance of gut flora, and imbalances are widespread in America. Whole body vibration can aid in promoting a healthy gut flora balance, because its effects strengthen the body and immune system. However, WBV can also aggravate gut flora imbalances when not used properly.

Natural health proponents have long stressed the importance of a healthy gut for overall health.[1-4] In the past, mainstream medicine was skeptical of this idea. Recently, however, there has been a surge of research and news articles regarding the link between gut flora imbalances and a wide range of health issues, including depression, anxiety, autism, digestive problems, weight gain, autoimmune system diseases, and allergies.[5-10] While gut flora generally stays in the gut, our digestive system is connected to the rest of our bodies in numerous ways, and inflammation and toxins produced by unwelcome gut dwellers can travel throughout the body.

Due to a perfect storm of factors, this gut fungal overgrowth has become an epidemic, especially in America. Poor nutrition weakens our immune systems and feeds fungal invaders with sugar. The overuse of antibiotics kills the beneficial bacteria in our guts, leaving an empty ecological niche with no competitors for space and food. Exposure to toxins and unrelenting stress can weaken our immune systems and bodies, leaving us susceptible to overgrowths of the wrong types of intestinal flora. One reason yogurt and other products with beneficial bacteria (probiotics) are currently so popular is because they repopulate the gut with health-promoting bacteria, thus helping to alleviate many different symptoms.

Whole body vibration can have a surprisingly big impact on gut flora. When used properly, its powerful detoxification effect, and many other health enhancing effects (see my book, *Whole Body Vibration: The Future of Good Health*), can strengthen the immune system, helping the body to fight detrimental bacteria. I often also recommend a program of probiotics, gentle natural antifungal agents, and dietary changes to go along with vibration. If you are experiencing chronic health issues, I recommend that you explore proper gut flora balance, as this is one of the most broadly effective approaches I use.

However, too much vibration, causing more detoxing than one's body can tolerate without a strain, can temporarily weaken one's immune system and its ability to fight bacteria and yeast. This can lead to a sudden increase of unwelcome gut flora with a corresponding flare-up of any symptoms caused by these invaders.

How much vibration is too much depends on the many factors affecting the strength of an individual's immune system, so it varies greatly from person to person. I recommend starting slowly and adjusting the amount as you become more aware of how your body reacts to vibration. Vibration will also help you become stronger, so you will likely be able to increase and do more over time, but even a very small amount of vibration can have a large and beneficial effect. The best approach is to do the amount that is right for your body.

Appendix 2

Live Cell Therapy

Live cell therapy is the use of live cell extracts, made from embryonic or fetal animal tissue, or the whole live cells to enhance the repair and regeneration of organs and tissue. Since these extracts are made from tissue at the fetal stage, a time when growth is accelerated, they are rich in molecules and nutrients that stimulate the growth of healthy new tissue. This type of nutrient rich "soup" naturally contains growth factors and tissue-signaling molecules, as well as some of the hottest new anti-aging molecules that have recently been discovered. With a history of approximately one century of use, this often overlooked therapy deserves closer examination.

There are many variations of "live cell therapy" that have many different names. Confusingly, the name "live cell therapy" is also sometimes used to refer to several different variations of cellular preparations and routes of administration, some of which do not actually contain live cells.

The name "live cell therapy" comes from the original development of this form of treatment by Dr. Niehans circa 1930. Actual live whole cells are still used in some injection forms of this therapy, but many preparations now consist of fetal cells that have been broken into their basic elements: enzymes, polypeptides, deoxyribonucleic acids, ribonucleic acids, and other basic organic substances. These components are believed to be variably, and sometimes highly, bio-available and bioactive.

I am going to limit my discussion here primarily to oral forms of "live cell therapy" in liquid preparations. (These do not contain whole live cells but rather extracts made from disrupted or broken cells.) I will include relevant observations that have been made using injections of whole live cells. Freeze-dried preparations are available, but freeze drying may denature (partially destroy) the complex molecules.

Injections of whole live cells are popular in other countries, but they are not legal in the US due to safety concerns. However, several million people have undergone live cell therapy injections over a period of about a hundred years, with only a low incidence reported of adverse reactions or clear causality. Concerns have been raised about immune system rejection of the injected cell material, and the animals used must be disease free. Exact risk/benefit ratios have not been established, but the reported anecdotal success and popularity of the method dictates a need for more testing and study. In the 1950s, almost two hundred hospitals in Germany were using this therapy, though its use has declined somewhat. Live cell therapy is still popular in Germany, however, and also in East Asian countries.

There is little dispute about the safety of oral forms of live cell therapy—it is similar safety-wise to ingesting raw animal flesh. Therefore, as long as care is taken to ensure that the animals are disease free, there is very little risk.

Sublingual liquid forms of the extract are held under the tongue for ten minutes before swallowing. Since veins and arteries are very close to the surface of the mucosal tissue under the tongue, there is variable but direct absorption into the bloodstream with this method. Another oral method employs encapsulation of live cell preparations to protect the complex molecules from the digestive process.

Unfortunately, allopathic medicine has tended to reject live cell therapy out of hand, because its claims of benefit have not been subjected to rigorous scientific research, and it has been argued that its proposed mechanisms of action are impossible. There has been very little double-blind, placebo-controlled modern research. Most of the current reports on the various forms of live cell therapy consist of observational studies. However, recent advances in medicine and science are lending some support to the underlying ideas behind live cell therapy, and the time is ripe for a further, more careful look at this novel method of treatment.

Organ Specific Healing?

Several theories have been proposed to explain the dramatic results of rapid healing that are sometimes reported with live cell therapy. There is much debate over the idea that these preparations are able to target specific organs. Research in Germany with injected cells tagged with radio-isotopic markers has supported the idea that live cell injections target diseased organs; for example, liver live cell molecules specifically migrating to and promoting healing in the recipient's liver. These results have not, however, been consistently reproduced.

One explanation proposed for this possible tissue "homing activity" is based in "bioenergetic concepts."[1] The idea is that a shared "vibrational" energy between similar cells (for example heart live cells and the recipient's heart cells) will lead to healing. This still-theoretical idea is rooted in the same concepts that underlie homeopathy—that similar substances can vibrate at similar frequencies, leading to "like cures like" healing phenomena.

Stephen Holt, MD, draws attention to the role that chemical signaling may play in live cell therapy in his latest book, *The Anti-Aging Triad: Calorie Restriction, Telomeres, Stem Cells*. He reports that scientists in Germany have measured increases in natural killer cells and other immune system cells within hours of live cell injections. Several other researchers have published papers discussing the complex and not yet fully understood nature of chemical signaling between cells in the body including foreign cells. These hypotheses provide peripheral support for this idea.

Dr. Holt also points out that early responses reported in the transplant of stem cells are unlikely to be due to the actual engraftment of the injected cells. A more likely mechanism is the signaling of body tissues by the embryonic cells. Dr. Holt has postulated that "the injection of foreign animal cells or their derivatives may actually cause mobilization of endogenous adult stem cells in the human recipient of live cell therapy."[2] Simply put, he is proposing the hypothesis that fetal animal cells may stimulate human stem cell activity.

Rejuvenating Mitochondria?

Meanwhile, one of the biggest areas of anti-aging research these days is in rejuvenating mitochondria, the powerhouses of energy production in our cells. Mitochondrial activity drops dramatically with age; by age eighty, they are functioning at only 4 percent of their normal youthful levels. While it is not clear why they fade as we age, this drop in energy production has been linked to everything from heart failure to neurodegeneration to just a lack of energy in daily life.

Attention has focused on a molecule called nicotinamide adenine dinucleotide (NAD), a key molecule for energy production within the mitochondria. In 2013, Harvard researcher David Sinclair published an article showing a nearly complete reversal of this drop in energy production in the mitochondria of older mice after just one week of injections of nicotinamide mononucleotide (NMN), a precursor of NAD; changes that are the equivalent of turning the energy production of a sixty-year-old human back to that of a twenty-year-old in one week. So far, however, only the mitochondria in the muscle cells of mice have been studied, not measures of other tissue health and strength—and no studies in humans. This is still very preliminary research.

Nevertheless, these results ignited a firestorm of attention, leading to the formation of several companies, some of them with Nobel Prize–winning scientists on their boards and all now researching and marketing supplements containing nicotinamide riboside (NR), another precursor to NAD.

For example, Elysium Health lists as advisors six Nobel laureates and more than fifteen other big names, such as the Mayo Clinic's Jim Kirkland and biotech pioneer Lee Hood.[3] Another, ChromaDex, has Roger Kornberg, who won the 2006 Nobel Prize in chemistry. One area of concern is affordability,* so more research in this area is needed.

NR and NMN are, in fact, vitamin B3 (niacin) precursors, and, as such, they are thought to be a natural part of the nutrient soup created with live cell extracts, which could account for some of the dramatic rejuvenating effects anecdotally reported with live cell therapy. This is not a far-fetched thought when you consider that our primary source of vitamin B3 is from ingesting animal flesh, and live cell extracts are made from embryonic or fetal animal tissues.

Potentially, a possibly lower number of vitamin B3 precursors in live cell extracts could be offset by the host of other cofactors and compounds that are combined with these prized molecules. This is a common effect when using supplements that are made from whole substances rather than using supplements that consist of an isolated nutrient. The reductionist approach of trying to determine an active ingredient, then taking large amounts of it in isolation, is a common approach in Western science and medicine, but it often backfires because essential cofactors are not there in sufficient quantities.

This is likely why the results of taking individual vitamins have been disappointing. Research published in the December 2013 *Annals of Internal Medicine* and other sources has shown, for example, that taking a multivitamin had little effect on heart problems or memory loss and wasn't tied to a longer life span.[4] However, eating fruits and vegetables, which are packed with vitamins and minerals, continues to be widely recognized as beneficial for heart and brain health, as well as the rest of the body, and linked to increased life expectancy.

---

*NMN is prohibitively expensive. According to some news reports, enough NMN to treat a person at the level that produced the one-week reversal of energy loss reported by Dr. Sinclair would cost $43,000 per day, while enough NR for the same result might cost around $100 per day. This still-prohibitive price is currently dealt with by lowering the amounts of NR, and NR-containing supplements are now available through several companies at a price in the range of anywhere from $7–$360 per month.

Studies have shown that the different results could be due to the many other nutrients found in the original fruits and vegetables that work in concert with the isolated vitamins. For example, Italian researchers in the Division of Human Nutrition at the University of Milan, Italy, found that vitamin C was not the only nutrient responsible for antioxidant protection. In oranges, vitamin C is part of a matrix involving many beneficial phytochemicals (for example, cyanidin-3-glucoside, flavanones, and carotenoids).[5]

Practical Issues

Live cell preparations can be made and introduced to the body in several different ways, and they can vary greatly in their purity, quality, effect, and cost. Some extracts are made from individual organs and used with the aim of targeting those organs. These extracts may provide intensive healing, but it is necessary to know which organs are damaged. Other preparations are more general and are hypothesized to be useful for nonspecific anti-aging stimulation.

The cost for oral live cell therapy supplements can range anywhere from forty to a thousand dollars per month, the length of treatment depending on the severity of the situation, and the effectiveness may vary greatly due to the quality of the preparation and type of product. Injections are currently not allowed in the US but can be obtained overseas. Unfortunately, in the US, live cell therapy is generally not covered by insurance.

While, live cell therapy can be expensive, it is still much less expensive than the heroic measures, such as joint replacements and organ transplants, that Western medicine typically offers. My personal belief is that we should devote much more time, energy, attention, and money to prevention and healing through natural health approaches. I have personally used a great deal of a liquid, sublingual, organ-specific form of live cell therapy for many struggling systems and organs in my body, and I can say that I saw dramatic and rapid results, sometimes within hours, when nothing else had worked.

In this country, we have the most technologically advanced medical system in the world, which serves a valuable and important purpose, especially in emergency situations, but it relies too heavily on drugs, surgery, and other radical interventions. Drugs often do not help your body truly heal, and they may have toxic side effects that often lead to further long-term health problems. Surgery carries risks and creates irreversible change and sometimes loss, when our body may have the ability to heal itself given the proper conditions.

We are lagging behind much of the world when it comes to the acceptance, use, and understanding of natural health approaches. We need to explore and use all avenues, especially natural health and energy medicine, to reach our highest state of health and well-being.

Notes

Foreword, by Burke Lennihan

1. P. S. Chikramane, D. Kalita, A. K. Suresh, S. G. Kane, and J. R. Bellare, "Why Extreme Dilutions Reach Non-Zero Asymptotes: A Nanoparticulate Hypothesis Based on Froth Flotation," *Langmuir*, November 2012, doi:10.1021/la303477s.

2. M. Enserink, "Newsmaker Interview: Luc Montagnier, French Nobelist Escapes 'Intellectual Terror' to Pursue Radical Ideas in China," *Science* 24 (December 2010): 1732, doi:10.1126 /science.330.6012.1732.

Chapter 1

1. H. L. Coulter, *Divided Legacy: The Conflict between Homeopathy and the American Medical Association* (Berkeley: North Atlantic Books, 1973).

2. Enserink, "Newsmaker Interview," 1732.

3. Paolo Bellavite and Signorini, *Emerging Science of Homeopathy: Complexity, Biodynamics, and Nanopharmacology* (Berkeley: North Atlantic Books, 2002), 170.

4. Ibid.

5. Dana Ullman, *The Homeopathic Revolution: Why Famous People and Cultural Heroes Choose Homeopathy* (Berkeley: North Atlantic Books, 2007), 102.

6. T. L. Bradford, *The Logic of Figures or Comparative Results of Homoeopathic and Other Treatments* (Philadelphia: Boiricke and Tafel, 1900).

7. Coulter, *Divided Legacy.*

8. Amy Lansky, *Impossible Cure: The Promise of Homeopathy* (Portola Valley, CA: R. L. Ranch Press, 2003), 4–5.

9. T. A. McCann, "Presidential Address," *Journal of the American Institute of Homeopathy* 14 (October 1921).

10. W. A. Dewey, "Homeopathy in Influenza: A Chorus of Fifty in Harmony," *Journal of the American Institute of Homeopathy* 14 (May 1921): 1038–1043.

11. "Medical Ethics," *New York Times,* June 1882, 4.

12. Coulter, *Divided Legacy.*

13. See https://en.wikipedia.org/wiki/World_Health_Organization_ranking_of_health_systems_in_2000.

14. M. Piolot, J. P. Fagot, S. Rivière, A. Fagot-Campagna, G. Debeugny, P. Couzigou, and F. Alla, "Homeopathy in France in 2011–2012 According to Reimbursements in the French National Health Insurance Database (SNIIRAM)" *Family Practice,* April 2015, doi:10.1093/fampra/cmv028.

15. A. Tuffs, "German Doctors and Politicians Disagree on Reimbursement for Homoeopathy," *British Medical Journal,* July 2010, doi:http://dx.doi.org/10.1136/bmj.c3902.

16. R. Prasad, "Homoeopathy Booming in India," *Lancet* 370, no. 9600 (2007): 1679–80, http://www.ncbi.nlm.nih.gov/pubmed/18035598.

17. Gudrun Bornhöft and Peter F. Matthiessen, *Homeopathy in Healthcare: Effectiveness, Appropriateness, Safety, Costs* (Goslar, Germany: Springer, 2011).

18. Gudrun Bornhöft, U. Wolf, K. von Ammon, M. Righetti, S. Maxion-Bergemann, S. Baumgartner, A. E. Thurneysen, P. F. Matthiessen, "Effectiveness, Safety, and Cost-Effectiveness of Homeopathy in General Practice: Summarized Health Technology Assessment," *Forschende Komplementärmedizin* 13, no. S2 (2006): 19–29.

19. Ullman, Dana. "The Swiss Government's Remarkable Report on Homeopathic Medicine." *Huffington Post,* September 18, 2013. http://www.huffingtonpost.com/dana-ullman/homeopathic-medicine-_b_1258607.html.

20. M. Frass, C. Dielacher, M. Linkesch, C. Endler, I. Muchitsch, E. Schuster, and A. Kaye, "Influence of Potassium Dichromate on Tracheal Secretions in Critically Ill Patients," *Chest*, March 2005.

21. Marsha Angell, *The Truth about Drug Companies* (New York: Random House, 2004).

22. R. Levi, "Science Is for Sale," *Skeptical Inquirer* 30, no. 4 (July/August 2006): 44–46.

23. "Americans Spent $33.9 Billion Out-of-Pocket on Complementary and Alternative Medicine," National Institutes of Health, nccih.nih.gov/news/2009/073009.htm.

24. Rustum Roy, William Tiller, Iris Bell, and M. R. Hoover. "The Structure of Liquid Water: Novel Insights from Materials Research; Potential Relevance to Homeopathy," *Materials Research Innovations* 9 (December 2005): 4.

25. Chikramane, et al., "Why Extreme Dilutions Reach Non-Zero Asymptotes."

26. Bellavite and Signorini, *Emerging Science of Homeopathy.*

27. Dana Ullman, "Luc Montagnier, Nobel Prize Winner, Takes Homeopathy Seriously," *Huffington Post,* October 2013, http://www.huffingtonpost.com/dana-ullman/luc-montagnier -homeopathy-taken-seriously_b_814619.html.

28. Martin Chaplin, Water Science and Structure website, www.lsbu .ac.uk/water/chaplin.html.

29. Roy, et al., 2005.

30. Enserink, "Newsmaker Interview," 1732.

31. Ullman, "Luc Montagnier, Nobel Prize Winner."

32. E. Davenas, F. Beauvais, J. Amara, et al. "Human Basophil Degranulation Triggered by Very Dilute Antiserum against IgE," *Nature* 333, no. 6176 (1988): 816–8.

33. B. D. Josephson, letter to the editor, *New Scientist*, November 1, 1997.

34. Peter Fisher, letter to the editor, "The End of the Benveniste Affair?" *British Homeopathic Journal* 88, no. 4 (1999).

35. Ullman, "Luc Montagnier, Nobel Prize Winner."

36. Samuel Hahnemann. *Organon of the Medical Art* (New Delhi, India: B. Jain Publishing, 2009).

37. Philip M. Bailey, MD, *Homeopathic Psychology: Personality Profiles of the Major Constitutional Remedies* (Berkeley: North Atlantic Books, 1995), xii.

38. H. G. Wells, *Mr. Brittling Sees It Through* (New York: MacMillan Co., 1916), 404.

Chapter 2

1. M. Ariizumi and A. Okada, "Effect of Whole Body Vibration on the Rat Brain Content of Serotonin and Plasma Corticosterone,"

European Journal of Applied Physiology and Occupational Physiology 52, no. 1 (1983): 15–9.

2. Gretchen Reynolds, "Jogging Your Brain," *New York Times* magazine, April 2012, 46.

3. Norman Shealy, MD, PhD, *Soul Medicine* (Santa Rosa, CA: Elite Books, 2006), 208–212.

4. Ibid., 16.

5. Richard Gerber, MD, *Vibrational Medicine,* 3rd ed. (Rochester, NY: Bear and Co., 2001), 53–56.

6. Shealy, *Soul Medicine,* 212.

7. Ibid., 213.

8. Ibid., 212.

9. Anne Trafton, "Synchronized Brain Waves Enable Rapid Learning: MIT Study Finds Neurons That Hum Together Encode New Information," MIT News Office, June 12, 2015, http://newsoffice.mit.edu/2014/synchronized-brain-waves-enable-rapid-learning-0612.

10. Ibid.

11. Ibid.

12. Keith DeOrio, MD. *Vibranetics: The Complete Whole Body Vibration Fitness Solution* (Santa Monica, CA: self-published, 2008), 31. (See www.drdeorio.com.)

Chapter 3

1. Roger Morrison, MD, *Desktop Guide to Keynotes and Confirmatory Symptoms* (Grass Valley, CA: Hahnemann Clinic Publishing, 1993), 259.

2. Morrison, *Desktop Guide to Keynotes,* 387.

3. Ibid., 33.

4. Ibid., 4.

5. Ibid., 291.

6. Ibid., 323–27.

7. Ibid., 40.

8. Bailey, *Homeopathic Psychology*, 46 (see chap. 1, n. 37).

9. Morrison, *Desktop Guide to Keynotes*, 89.

10. Ibid., 256.

11. Ibid., 257.

12. Ibid., 44.

Chapter 4

1. Morrison, *Desktop Guide to Keynotes*, 83.

2. Ibid., 84.

3. Bailey, *Homeopathic Psychology*, 46.

4. Morrison, *Desktop Guide to Keynotes*, 323–26.

5. Ibid., 55–57.

6. Bailey, *Homeopathic Psychology*, 254.

7. Ibid., 254–55.

8. Morrison, *Desktop Guide to Keynotes*, 292–95.

9. Ibid., 330.

10. Ibid., 307.

Chapter 5

1. Morrison, *Desktop Guide to Keynotes,* 124 (see chap. 3, n. 1).

2. Ibid., 401.

3. Ibid., 404.

4. Ibid., 169.

5. Ibid.

6. Ibid., 255.

7. Ibid., 259.

8. Ibid., 273.

9. Ibid., 275.

10. Ibid., 381.

11. Robin Murphy, ND, *Homeopathic Medical Repertory* (Pagosa Springs, CO: Hahnemann Academy of North America, 1993), 669.

12. Morrison, *Desktop Guide to Keynotes,* 200.

13. Ibid.

Chapter 6

1. Morrison, *Desktop Guide to Keynotes,* 216.

2. Bailey, *Homeopathic Psychology,* 101 (see chap. 1, n. 37).

3. Ibid.

4. Morrison, *Desktop Guide to Keynotes,* 376–77.

5. Ibid., 376–78.

6. Ibid., 207.

7. Ibid., 256.

8. Ibid., 257.

9. Bailey, *Homeopathic Psychology,* 293.

10. Morrison, *Desktop Guide to Keynotes,* 344.

11. Bailey, *Homeopathic Psychology,* 296.

12. Morrison, *Desktop Guide to Keynotes,* 344.

Chapter 7

1. Morrison, *Desktop Guide to Keynotes,* 39–44.

2. Bailey, *Homeopathic Psychology,* 16.

3. Morrison, *Desktop Guide to Keynotes,* 387.

4. W. Boericke, MD, *Homoeopathic Materia Medica and Repertory* (New Delhi, India: B. Jain Publishers, Ltd., 2004), 516–17.

5. Robin Murphy, ND. *Nature's Materia Medica,* 3rd ed. (Blacksburg, VA: Lotus Health Institute, 2006), 1524–27.

6. Morrison, *Desktop Guide to Keynotes,* 111.

7. Ibid., 50–51.

8. Ibid., 258–59.

9. Murphy, *Nature's Materia Medica,* 283.

10. Bailey, *Homeopathic Psychology,* 16.

Epilogue

1. W. M. Osler, "Physics and Physicians as Depicted in Plato," *New England Journal of Medicine* 128, no. 7 (1893).

Appendix 1

1. Bernard Jensen, *Dr. Jensen's Guide to Better Bowel Care* (New York: Avery/Penguin Putnam Inc., 1999).

2. Friedhelm Kirchfeld and Wade Boyle, *Nature Doctors: Pioneers in Naturopathic Medicine* (Portland, OR: Medicina Biologica, 1994).

3. William Crook, *The Yeast Connection: A Medical Breakthrough* (CA: Crown Publishing Group, 1994).

4. John Parks Trowbridge, MD, and Morton Walker, DPM, *The Yeast Syndrome* (New York: Bantam Books, 1985).

5. Kevin Jiang, "Gut Bacteria That Protect Against Food Allergies Identified," *Science Life,* August 25, 2014, http://sciencelife .uchospitals.edu/2014/08/25/gut-bacteria-that-protect-against -food-allergies-identified.

6. Rob Stein, "Mix of Gut Microbes May Play Role in Crohn's Disease," National Public Radio, March 12, 2014, http://www .npr.org/sections/health-shots/2014/03/12/289041150/mix-of -gut-microbes-may-play-role-in-crohns-disease.

7. Michaeleen Doucleff, "How Modern Life Depletes Our Gut Microbes, National Public Radio, April 21, 2015, http://www.npr .org/sections/goatsandsoda/2015/04/21/400393756/how-modern -life-depletes-our-gut-microbes.

8. Claudia Wallis, "How Gut Bacteria Help Make Us Fat and Thin," *Scientific American* 310, no. 6 (June 1, 2014), http://www .scientificamerican.com/article/how-gut-bacteria-help-make-us-fat -and-thin.

9. Melinda Wenner Moyer, "Gut Bacteria May Play a Role in Autism," *Scientific American* 25, no. 5 (August 14, 2014) http://www .scientificamerican.com/article/gut-bacteria-may-play-a-role-in -autism.

10. Carolyn Gregoire, "The Surprising Link between Gut Bacteria and Anxiety," *Huffington Post*, April 1, 2015, http://www.huffington post.com/2015/01/04/gut-bacteria-mental-healt_n_6391014.html.

Appendix 2

1. Stephen Holt, MD, *The Anti-Aging Triad: Calorie Restriction, Telomeres, Stem Cells* (Bloomington, IN: AuthorHouse, 2011), 268, 271.

2. Ibid., 278–79.

3. See http://www.elysiumhealth.com/team.

4. Brenda Goodman, "Experts: Don't Waste Your Money on Multivitamins; Three Studies Find the Supplements Don't Help Extend Life or Ward Off Heart Disease and Memory Loss," WebMD, http://www.webmd.com/vitamins-and-supplements/news /20131216/experts-dont-waste-your-money-on-multivitamins.

5. S. Guarnieri, P. Riso, M. Porrini, "Orange Juice vs. Vitamin C: Effect on Hydrogen Peroxide–Induced DNA Damage in Mononuclear Blood Cells," *British Journal of Nutrition* 97, no. 4 (2007):639–43.

Resources, Suggested Reading, and Additional References

Resources

Becky Chambers, natural health practitioner, BS, MEd
   Vibrant Health
   www.BCVibrantHealth.com

Homeopathic Organizations

American Institute of Homeopathy
   www.homeopathyusa.org

European Council for Classical Homeopathy (ECCH)
   www.homeopathy-ecch.org
   Information and referrals to professional homeopaths in Europe

Homeopathic Educational Services
   www.homeopathic.com
   Dana Ullman's website with information and further resources

National Center for Homeopathy
   www.homeopathic.org

North American Society of Homeopaths
www.homeopathy.org

www.homeopathy-cures.com/search.html
A referral list for classical homeopaths in the US and Canada

www.homeopathicdirectory.com
Offers referrals to all certified homeopaths in the United States
and Canada

www.homeopathyhome.com
A comprehensive and international guide to homeopathy that has
links to many other resources and websites

Suggested Reading

Introductory Self-Care Homeopathic Books

Bailey, Philip. *Homeopathic Psychology: Personality Profiles of the Major Constitutional Remedies*. Berkeley: North Atlantic Books, 1995.

Castro, Miranda. *The Complete Homeopathy Handbook: A Guide to Everyday Health Care*. New York: St. Martin's Press, 1991.

Coulter, Catherine. *Nature and Human Personality: Homoeopathic Archetypes*. Berkeley Springs, WV: Ninth House Publishing, 2002.

Cummings, Stephen, and Dana Ullman. *Everybody's Guide to Homeopathic Medicines: Safe and Effective Medicines for You and Your Family,* 3rd rev. ed. Los Angeles: J. P. Tarcher, 1997.

Grossinger, Richard. *Homeopathy: The Great Riddle*. Berkeley: North Atlantic Books, 1998.

Hershoff, Asa. *Homeopathic Remedies: A Quick and Easy Guide to Common Disorders and Their Homeopathic Treatments*. New York: Avery, 2000.

Lansky, Amy. *Impossible Cure: The Promise of Homeopathy*. Portola Valley, CA: R. L. Ranch Press, 2004.

Lennihan, Burke. *Your Natural Medicine Cabinet: A Practical Guide to Drug-Free Remedies for Common Ailments.* Cambridge, MA: GreenHealing Press, 2012.

Lockie, Andrew, and Nicola Geddes. *Complete Guide to Homeopathy.* New York: D. Kindersley, 2000.

Panos, Maesimund B., and Jane Heimlich. *Homeopathic Medicine at Home: Natural Remedies for Everyday Ailments and Minor Injuries.* Los Angeles: J. P. Tarcher, 1980.

Shalts, Edward. *The American Institute of Homeopathy Handbook for Parents.* San Francisco: Jossey-Bass, 2005.

More Advanced and Specialized Self-Care Homeopathic Books

Castro, Miranda. *Homeopathy for Pregnancy, Birth, and Your Baby's First Year.* New York: St. Martin's Press, 1997.

Chappell, Peter. *Emotional Healing with Homeopathy.* Berkeley: North Atlantic Books, 2003.

Hamilton, Don. *Homeopathic Care for Cats and Dogs.* Berkeley: North Atlantic Books, 2003.

Hershoff, Asa. *Homeopathy for Musculoskeletal Healing.* Berkeley: North Atlantic Books, 1996.

Lalor, Liz. *A Homeopathic Guide to Partnership and Compatibility.* Berkeley: North Atlantic Books, 2004.

Moskowitz, Richard. *Homeopathic Medicine for Pregnancy and Childbirth.* Berkeley: North Atlantic Books, 1992.

Reichenberg-Ullman, Judyth, and Robert Ullman. *Prozac Free: Homeopathic Medicines for Depression, Anxiety, and Other Mental and Emotional Problems.* Berkeley: North Atlantic Books.

————. *Ritalin-Free Kids*. New York: Three Rivers, 1996.

————. *Whole Woman Homeopathy: The Comprehensive Guide to Treating PMS, Menopause, Cystitis, and Other Problems Naturally and Effectively*. Rocklin, CA: Prima Publishing, 2000.

Homeopathic Research

Bellavite, Paolo, and Andrea Signorini. *The Emerging Science of Homeopathy: Complexity, Biodynamics, and Nanopharmacology*. Berkeley: North Atlantic Books, 2002.

Boyd, Linn. *A Study of the Simile in Medicine*. Philadelphia: Boericke and Tafel, 1936.

Coulter, H. L. *Divided Legacy: A History of the Schism in Medical Thought*, vols. 1–4. Washington, DC: Wehawken, 1975–1994.

Gray, Bill. *Homeopathy: Science or Myth?* Berkeley: North Atlantic Books, 2000.

Jonas, Wayne B., and Jennifer Jacobs. *Healing with Homeopathy*. New York: Warner, 1996.

Ullman, Dana. *Homeopathic Family Medicine*. https://www.homeopathic.com/cms-global/shoppingcart/ViewProduct.do?productId=227. Subscription e-book.

Candida Yeast

Chaitow, Leon. *Candida Albicans: Could Yeast Be Your Problem?* Rochester, VT: Healing Arts Press, 1998.

Crook, William. *The Yeast Connection: A Medical Breakthrough*. Berkeley: Crown Publishing Group, 1994.

Trowbridge, John Parks, and Morton Walker. *The Yeast Syndrome.* New York: Bantam Books, 1985.

Wunderlich, Ray Jr., and Dwight Kalita. *The Candida Yeast Syndrome.* New York: McGraw-Hill, 1998.

Additional References

Antzoulatos, E. G., E. K. and Miller. "Increases in Functional Connectivity between the Prefrontal Cortex and Striatum during Category Learning." *Neuron* 83 (2014): 216–225.

Bornhoft, Gudrun, and Peter F. Matthiessen. "Homeopathy in Healthcare: Effectiveness, Appropriateness, Safety, Costs." Goslar, Germany: Springer, 2011.

Bornhöft, Gudrun, U. Wolf, K. von Ammon, M. Righetti, S. Maxion-Bergemann, S. Baumgartner, A. E. Thurneysen, and P.F. Matthiessen. "Effectiveness, Safety, and Cost-Effectiveness of Homeopathy in General Practice: Summarized Health Technology Assessment." *Forschende Komplementärmedizin* 13, no. S2 (2006): 19–29.

Bouchayer, F. "Alternative Medicines: A General Approach to the French Situation." *Complimentary Medical Research* 4 (1990): 4–8.

Chambers, Becky. *Whole Body Vibration: The Future of Good Health.* Charlottesville, VA: Quartet Books, 2013.

Elia, V., S. Baiano, I. Duro, E. Napoli, M. Niccoli, and L. Nonatelli. "Permanent Physio-Chemical Properties of Extremely Diluted Aqueous Solutions of Homeopathic Medicines." *Homeopathy* 93 (2004): 144–150.

Elia, V., M. and Niccoli. "Thermodynamics of Extremely Diluted Aqueous Solutions." *Annals of the New York Academy of Sciences* 879 (1999): 241–48.

Linde, K., N. Clausius, G. Ramirez, et al. "Are the Clinical Effects of Homoeopathy Placebo Effects? A Meta-Analysis of Placebo-Controlled Trials." *Lancet* 350 (September 20, 1997): 834–43.

Perlmutter, David. *Brain Maker: The Power of Gut Microbes to Heal and Protect Your Brain—for Life*. New York: Little, Brown and Company, 2015.

Poitevin, B. "Integrating Homoeopathy in Health Systems." *Bulletin of the World Health Organization* 77, no. 2 (1999): 160–66.

Sardi, Bill. "Longevinex Is Best Way to Duplicate Age-Reversing Effects Produced in Recent Animal Laboratory Study." Resveratrol News.com, December 24, 2013. http://www.resveratrolnews.com /longevinex-best-way-to-duplicate-age-reversing-effects-produced -in-recent-animal-laboratory-study/862.

Stipp, David. "Beyond Resveratrol: The Anti-Aging NAD Fad." *Scientific American*, March 11, 2015. http://blogs.scientificamerican.com /guest-blog/beyond-resveratrol-the-anti-aging-nad-fad.

Wharton, R., and G. Lewith, "Complementary Medicine and the General Practitioner." *British Medical Journal* 292 (1986): 1490–1500.

Brain Synchronization

Abraha, I., F. Trotta, J. M. Rimland, A. Cruz-Jentoft, I. Lozano-Montoya, R. L. Soiza, V. Pierini, et al. "Efficacy of Non-Pharmacological Interventions to Prevent and Treat Delirium in Older Patients: A Systematic Overview. The SENATOR project ONTOP Series." *PLOS ONE* 10, no. 6 (June 2015). doi:10.1371 /journal.pone.0123090.

Danilenko, K. V., and I. A. Ivanova. "Dawn Simulation vs. Bright Light in Seasonal Affective Disorder: Treatment Effects and Subjective Preference." *Journal of Affective Disorders* 180 (July 15, 2015): 87–9. doi:10.1016/j.jad.2015.03.055.

da Silva, V. F., A. P. Ribeiro, V. A. Dos Santos, A. E. Nardi, A. L. King, and M. R. Calomeni. "Stimulation by Light and Sound: Therapeutics Effects in Humans: Systematic Review." *Clinical Practice and Epidemiology in Mental Health* 11 (June 26, 2015): 150–54. doi:10.2174/1745017901511010150.

Petrovsky, D., P. Z. Cacchione, and M. George. "Review of the Effect of Music Interventions on Symptoms of Anxiety and Depression in Older Adults with Mild Dementia." *International Psychogeriatrics* 27, no. 10 (April 29, 2015): 1–10. doi:10.1017/S1041610215000393.

Raglio, A., C. Galandra, L. Sibilla, F. Esposito, F. Gaeta, F. Di Salle, L. Moro, et al. "Effects of Active Music Therapy on the Normal Brain: fMRI Based Evidence." *Brain Imaging and Behavior,* April 7, 2015. http://www.ncbi.nlm.nih.gov/pubmed/25847861.

Schwartz, R. S., and J. Olds. "The Psychiatry of Light." *Harvard Review of Psychiatry* 23, no. 3 (May/June 2015): 188–94. doi:10.1097/HRP.0000000000000078.

Shealy, C. N. "The Reality of EEG and Neurochemical Responses to Photostimulation: Part I. In *Light Years Ahead: The Illustrated Guide to Full Spectrum and Colored Light in Mindbody Healing,* edited by Brian Breiling. Berkeley: Celestial Arts Press, 1996.

———. "The Reality of EEG and Neurochemical Responses to Photostimulation: Part II. In *Light Years Ahead: The Illustrated Guide to Full Spectrum and Colored Light in Mindbody Healing,* edited by Brian Breiling. Berkeley: Celestial Arts Press, 1996.

———, R. K. Cady, D. C. Veehoff, M. Burnetti-Atwell, R. Houston, and R. H. Cox. "Effects of Color Photostimulation upon Neurochemicals and Neurohormones." *Journal of Neurological and Orthopaedic Medicine and Surgery* 17, no. 1 (1996): 95–96.

————, T. L. Smith, P. Thomlinson, and W. A. Tiller. "A Double-Blind EEG Response Test for a Supposed Electromagnetic Field-Neutralizing Device. Part I: Via the Clinician Expertise Procedure." *Subtle Energies and Energy Medicine* 9, no. 3, 231–45.

Sun J., and W. Chen. "Music Therapy for Coma Patients: Preliminary Results." *European Review for Medical and Pharmacological Sciences* 19, no. 7 (April 2015): 1209–18. http://www.ncbi.nlm.nih.gov/pubmed/25912580.

◣◖◢

About the Author

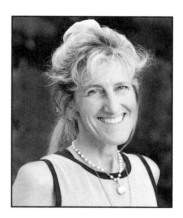

Becky Chambers is a natural health practitioner, teacher, author, and the president and owner of Vibrant Health, where she specializes in homeopathy and the breakthrough body, mind, and energy therapy of whole body vibration. Becky is one of the most experienced independent experts in whole body vibration in the United States. Her book, *Whole Body Vibration: The Future of Good Health,* has been the best-selling book in the US on this revolutionary technology since it was first published in 2013. Becky has since published a second book, *Homeopathy Plus Whole Body Vibration.*

Becky has a bachelor of science degree in biology from the University of Massachusetts, a master's in education from Lesley College, and she graduated from Clayton College of Natural Health in 2003 with a graduate degree in natural health, specializing in homeopathy.

She has spent the last twenty-five years discovering powerful new energy therapies that have led to a transformation of her life on every level. She has also published a memoir (not currently in print), *Beyond the Great Abyss: A True Story of Transformation through Natural Health Breakthroughs*.

Please visit her website at www.BCVibrantHealth.com.